Unlock The Secret To Weight Loss Victory! Stop Dumb Diets; Eat Food You Like!

A Simple System, You Eat The Foods You Like And Still Lose Weight

I0440007

Introduction

This book brings a new, and very practical approach to losing weight that's achievable by anyone. Rather than proposing a diet, extolling the virtues of exercise, or telling you what to eat, I explain the real issues that stand in everyone's path for weight loss, and more importantly I also explain some simple, and proven, methods for resolving those issues. I also explain the reason we continually drift from our path to weight loss victory, and how to find, and take advantage of, your secret; knowing what to do with that secret will make all the difference in the world, for your weight loss success. My goal is to clear the path to the elusive goal of long-term weight loss, and help you leave the ranks of the "Yo-Yo Diet Club".

I'm well aware that there's a large amount of weight loss material already written, in fact, over the years, I've read an awful lot of it myself. I'm not saying that what's been written in the past is wrong, but most of it just skirts the real issues, and offers few practical long-term solutions. This book is for everyone that's been fighting weight loss battles, as I've done for years. Everyone wants to finally get off the endless road of yo-yo dieting, and have the pleasure of achieving long-term sensible weight; who among us doesn't wish for that?

I'm now in my 70s, and first started to deal with being a little "husky" at about ten, so I've suffered, off and on, for over 60 years with this "overweight nightmare". Over the years I've gotten really tired of listening to so-called "weight loss gurus", who've promoted every kind of imaginable diet, "magic" pill, virtually every type of exercise equipment, diet food regime and more.

Honestly, I've never been able to relate to those opportunistic groups that seemed much more interested in selling a product, member-ships or some other "instant gratification" system for weight loss. Instinctively, I've always known that long-term weight loss was going to require long-term changes, but I was never able to successfully wrap my arms around the heart of that process until recently.

I started my first successful business in the early 1960s, and a number of other successful businesses followed through the years, I was successfully elected to public office, I became a corporate executive for a national company, and more. The reason I mention this, is because I realized that most people who have seen success in business, have also had to make some challenging long-term changes in their life. I reasoned that perhaps the time-tested methods used in business, if adapted properly, would also be hugely beneficial for the achievement of long-term weight loss. After a few years of experimenting with this concept, I felt that what I learned could be extremely beneficial to others, and I'm writing this book to share what I've learned. You'll see after reading this book that anyone who truly wants to change their weight situation in life, can do so by working his or her way through the simple steps that I lay out.

It is my hope that you'll find this book to be useful, and a roadmap for your successful long-term weight loss journey. The book is not an elitist weight loss system being promoted by some food or fitness "guru", nor is it a scientific journal of any kind; but, rather it's a fresh new weight loss perspective based on my life-long personal experiences, along with the utilization of proven business techniques. I did my best to keep it simple and easy to understand, so that you could quickly start using it on your own. It's my belief that in order for your weight loss program to be truly successful, it needs to be individually designed by you. Additionally, it's design must allow for the eating the foods that you enjoy the most, and that fit in smoothly with your individual life circumstances, abilities and desires. This is the only kind of plan that can garner the personal ownership, and acceptance, required in order to sustain long-term success.

I start this book by telling a little bit of personal background, and some of the different diets that I've tried over the years. The heart of this book, however, focuses on the steps that you can very easily take, and how they will get you started in the correct weight loss direction. For many, these steps may be life changing as they can also be applied to other areas of your life as well, but that's not the point here, as these steps are what's absolutely required for long-term weight loss success. I also want to be clear about the fact that although you may not currently be familiar with every step, they are not complicated and they're absolutely achievable by everyone.

I've laid out this information in a fashion that makes it easily implemented by you, and can easily be fit into whatever personal situation, or schedule, that you may have. The one consistent theme that carries throughout this entire book is that in order for your long-term weight loss plan to be successful, it's absolutely imperative that it be fully accepted, and embraced by you. Your plan needs to be designed by you to fit your desires and your individual life pattern, and that's why the guidelines for your plan will also be established by you. Anything less than that is simply a plan designed by someone else whose trying to give you what they think will work for you, and we've all tried that kind of plan, without much success.

If you're up for the challenge of making a positive weight loss change in your life, you'll find a lot of very useful information in what you're about to read, and you'll enjoy it too. This book is the "real deal", and everything in this book is absolutely achievable by you, no matter who you are. You must just be willing to follow these concepts, and take leadership for your future self.

Table Of Contents

Unlock The Secret To Weight Loss Victory!
Stop Dumb Diets; Eat Food You Like!
by Lyle T. Gilbertson

Section I
My Story

I want to begin with some history of my weight loss issues, as I feel that it's likely that many of you will identify with some of what I have to share. I know that many of you have weight loss stories far more grievous than my own. My point with these few paragraphs is simply to let you know that we're all in this same boat together, and my ultimate goal is to bring some practical reality, to the insanity of the yo-yo dieting that seems to go on continually, for all of us.

I've struggled with my weight, ever since I can remember. It's not that I was overly heavy as a youth; I was sort of what you called Husky. What that really means, is that I was probably somewhere from 10 to 15 pounds overweight throughout many of those years. I was always aware of my extra weight because I couldn't run quite as fast as some of the other kids, or jump as high. Still I could play sports, had lots of friends and pretty much had a wonderful time in my growing up years.

In that my youth took place mostly in the 1940's, and 1950's, a lot of things have changed since then. Generally speaking, obesity was not as prevalent in those years as it is today. I suppose that my 10 or 15 pounds of overweight might be considered fairly normal today, though at the time I always felt that I was a little bit "pudgy". As I look back on it, I think that our family had reasonably good eating habits. We ate lots of fish, salads, soups and some red meats. With that said, it was also normal in those years to coat fish, or chicken, with a flour batter and fry it in oil. That wasn't the case all the time, as I can recall having broiled fish, broiled steak, and a large variety of different types of salads, but greasy fried food was also common.

I can't honestly say that sweets were a major part of our diet, at least it didn't seem that way. The fact is, however, that there was always bread and jelly on the table, peanut butter and jelly sandwiches in my lunch box, pies cakes or cookies for dessert, and occasionally there was candy around the house. The breakfast norm seemed to be Bacon and eggs, pancakes with syrup, or cereal with whole milk and sugar on it, (there was always a sugar bowl on the table). A large amount of whole milk was always available, and I can never remember there not being cookies in the pantry. So in retrospect, although the eating habits in our household seemed to be much the same as those of my friends, it's pretty clear to me now, that I grew up eating a diet fairly heavy in both fats and sugars.

At 17, I went away to college. In the first two years of college, I either ate at the college commons or at the fraternity house. Like most kids off to college, I felt that the food wasn't as good as what I was used to at home. Nevertheless, as I look back on it, the balance of the foods, fats and sweets, was pretty much the same as it had been for me through all my years to that point. Of course, now I was away from home, and joined other college friends in snacking at local hangouts, and buying food from the ever-present vending machines.

During my last two years at college, I shared an apartment with other students, and we often did our own cooking. I can't honestly say that our cooking was a dietary improvement. We ate lots of starchy foods, stuff we liked, and ate out at many of the cheap dives that fed you a lot of food for not much money. Although I rarely went to church during those college years, many of my friends and I would often go to one of the many church pancake breakfasts, which were so prevalent in college towns. At the time I didn't under-stand that the congregation really appreciated young college kids coming to hang out around the church, but we just loved the free breakfasts with unlimited pancakes, syrup and sausage. Not really very healthy, but the price was right, we always ate a lot, had fun, and as I said, the congregation always welcomed us back.

Soon after college I was married, and began a life of home-cooked meals. I can't really say that the food, or dietary habits changed much through those early years. As the years moved on, however, the food grew richer, and the quantities greater, as our family became a little more affluent. Now that I had a much less active lifestyle as a businessperson, the richer foods tied to less activity started to take its toll in terms of additional weight.

At nearly age 30, I realized that my current weight of about 235 pounds had become excessive. To put that into perspective, I was six foot one, and about 195 when I graduated from college. So it was then, at about age 30 that I first decided to do something about that excess 40 pounds. It was about 1968, well before anyone had ever heard of Dr. Adkins, or the Atkins Diet. But, one day, someone gave me a mimeograph copy of a diet plan that basically consisted of eliminating pretty much all carbohydrates from your diet. Now, I don't necessarily embrace this diet, as I'm not personally sure that skipping carbohydrates, and allowing yourself to eat fatty foods, is wise, healthy or even useful as a means for long-term weight loss. Nevertheless I gave this diet a try, which required me to religiously avoid eating breads, sugars, potatoes, pasta and other starchy foods, while still eating meats, cheeses, fish, poultry and etc.

All this was a number of years ago of course, so it's hard to remember specifically, but I don't recall having any particular hardships on this diet, other than minor inconveniences when eating in restaurants. The fact is, over a period of about six months I lost about 45 pounds, and actually had to retrain myself to go back to eating regularly so that I would stop losing weight. Unfortunately, what I called eating regularly has not appeared to be overly beneficial to me, throughout the years. In the many years since then, my weight has continued to fluctuate up and down, mostly between about 225 pounds to as high as 265 pounds (on two separate occasions). Within the past year and a half, by regulating the food that I ate, I was able to drop my weight from 265 down to 235. Unfortunately, however, in the last six or nine months I somehow lost my focus, and the weight started to climb again. But, this time I realized that this past weight loss effort was significantly different; I had approached it differently, and I now began to see that there truly was hope for long-term weight loss success, and that over time I was going to be able to maintain my weight at around the 190 pound range that I want to achieve.

So there is a little history of where I've come from through the years, weight wise, and where I am today. My whole point in writing this history of my past weight loss, and weight gain, is simply to illustrate that my issues with maintaining a stable healthy weight is very likely much like your own experience, and not at all like many of the so called "weight loss gurus" that have never been overweight a day in their lives.

As I said earlier, I want to share with you some important things that I've discovered in this past year or so, including how we must go about examining our individual weight loss situations. We'll also have to adjust our perspective on a few things, and then keep those changes rock solid throughout the rest of our lives. But most importantly this book will show you simple and workable ways to make these permanent changes. I will outline the complete weight loss and weight stabilization plan that's working for me, and that I know can also work for you. As you read through this book, you will see that I've merged many business development concepts with sensible, and easily manageable, weight loss approaches. If you're serious about managing your weight for the long-term, then you'll find that this program is one that's practical, simple and easily executable by you; it's a program that will work, plain and simple.

Section II
Weight Loss Systems That I've Tried

Before we go on to any new weight loss ideas, I'd like to review some of the weight loss plans that I've tried in the past. I'm sure that you've had your share of weight loss plans too; I'd guess that between all of us we've tried an awful lot of different things. Through the years, off and on, I've personally attempted numerous systems for weight loss. Although I've made progress from time to time, I was never able to fully achieve my long-term objective. Of course, you have your own weight loss history and experiences, and going forward I believe it's going to be helpful for you to review what you've attempted in the past, so that you'll be able to analyze what worked for you, and what fell short. My objective, in sharing these weight loss experiences, and systems, is hopefully to let you observe that we've all been struggling with the same kinds of issues.

"The No Carbohydrate Diet"

As I described earlier, my first serious attempt at weight loss was when I was around 28 years old, and found that I was now carrying about 40 extra pounds of fat. That's when someone handed me that mimeographed, no carbohydrate, diet plan. This is the diet I described earlier that basically eliminated carbohydrates, and said that it was okay to eat fatty foods such as cheese, burgers (without bread) and other such foods. Although I actually lost substantial weight after six months or so, I unfortunately later gained it back again.

At this point in my life I was not overly focused on dieting, and although I was happy to lose the weight, I had little idea as to why this diet worked for me, or whether or not it was beneficial health wise. As the years passed, I've learned a lot more about different food types, and how they affect me. I've actually returned to this type of diet a few more times over the years. My personal observation of how it affected me personally, is as

10

follows: (1) I still have no knowledge as to the overall affect of this type of diet on my health, but I would suspect that it's long-term health benefits could seriously be questioned, based on what I now feel is a lack of being a balanced diet. (2) My recollection is that this diet tended to make me somewhat constipated. (3) Although I've never been a person who has been particularly addicted to sweets, pastry or breads, I do recall that being on this diet tended to make me start to crave those sweets, and the starchy foods that I was not eating.

Overall my experience with this type of diet seemed fairly acceptable to me, but any weight that I lost tended to come back fairly quickly as I returned to what I felt was a normal diet. It's also possible that when I did return to eating "normally", I may have overreacted some, and allowed myself to be a little extra indulgent in eating those sweet, and starchy foods that I had been lacking.

Fasting

Some years later, when I was in about my mid-thirties or so, I read a book on dieting by fasting. It was fairly convincing, at least enough so that I thought I'd like to try it, and so that's what I did. I seem to have lost track of the actual book so I can't tell you exactly how the fasting took place. But, as I recall I started with a few days of fruit juice, then a couple days of watered down fruit juice, then followed by 10 days, or maybe two weeks, of complete fasting and drinking nothing but water. In the beginning I thought that I'd never make it very far, but as it turned out I actually didn't find it too difficult. At that point, as I recall, I went back to a few days of the fruit juice followed by easing into a simple balanced diet that was supposed to now be my life long eating regiment. The fact was I did lose weight rather dramatically during those first few weeks, and for whatever reason continued to lose some additional weight even after I'd started eating in a normal fashion. Soon, however, my old "normal" eating habits resumed, and the weight loss was not sustained.

I recall from my original reading about this diet that was not recommended for people over 40. Personally, I'm not at all sure that following this kind of diet regiment is either healthy, or makes any sense for anyone. I'm sure there are many people who might disagree with that, and who believe that so-called "body cleansing", is very healthy behavior. Since my one time try with this "fasting diet" I've never tried it again except for those few times that I was required to fast prior to a medical procedure. Fasting might be a wonderful thing, but my personal opinion is that if a person wants to follow a fasting diet, it should only be done with a physician's supervision, and/or recommendation.

The "French" Diet

When I was in my early 50's a friend of mine recommended a book called "Dine Out And Lose Weight", by Michel Montignac. In the late 1980s this book was a bestseller in France, under the name "Comment maignir en faisant des respas d'affaires". It was in the early 1990s that this book was published, and republished in English, and although I don't think it ever became a US bestseller, I found this to be one of the most informative books on dieting that I'd read. Although I have the 1991 paperback edition of this book, I have no reason to believe that the later editions are much different, other than being updated with some new diets. Unfortunately, I suspect that this book may be out of print, but there may be a few new copies, as well some used copies, available at both www.Amazon.com and www.Abebooks.com. A fast way to locate this book is with the ISBN: 2906236179, and I highly recommend this book for anyone interested in learning more about a somewhat unique, and very interesting approach to foods.

In many ways the diet outlined in "Dine Out And Lose Weight", is similar to the "Atkins Diet", and to the "no carbohydrate diet", except that it does include carbohydrates. The book goes into great detail explaining the history of French diets, and how the French seem to have been able to keep their weight naturally under control through the years, with foods that we normally think of as being "fattening". It also explains the differences between simple carbohydrates (the "bad" carbohydrates like sugars, most breads, and other starchy foods), and complex carbohydrates (the "good" carbohydrates like whole cereals, brown rice, beans, fruit and etc.). Unfortunately, my explanation is very much an over simplification of the "Dine Out And Lose Weight" diet concept, as it goes into much more detail and includes in-depth explanations as to both the benefits, and the drawbacks, of multiple food types, and how these food types interact with each other.

Personally, when I initially tried the "Dine Out And Lose Weight", I lost weight, and felt really good about the eating habits that it tried to teach me. As has happened numerous other times in my life, I tended to drift away from following their diet regiment, even though it was probably the one of the better diet plan that I'd found to this point in my life. With that said, however, I can tell you that to this day the book "Dine Out And Lose Weight" has taught me to understand food differently, and this book's underlying principles still stick with me. Because of this, I now have a much clearer understanding of the different food types, how they possibly interact with one another, and how those different food types will likely affect me.

Hypnosis

I first tried hypnosis, as a means for weight loss, when I was in my early 50s. I went to a professional hypnotherapist, who had a wonderful comfortable setting along with a very good track record for helping people with weight loss. I had already read a considerable amount about hypnosis, and its use as a vehicle for weight loss. I felt that the concept was very viable, as I still do, and I was anxious to try it.

13

Unfortunately, my first experience at weight loss with a hypnotherapist turned out to be a failure, simply because it turns out that for whatever reason, I am not a person who is very susceptible to being hypnotized. Still, however, I continued to experiment with some of the recorded weight loss programs that are intended to help you subliminally, as you sleep. Because of my experience in business, I understood the value putting the proper messages firmly into the subconscious mind; it's truly a powerful means for changing behaviors.

Still, after all of these attempts, I had little or nothing to show in terms of changed behavior that would help me with my weight loss journey. Let's be clear, I believe that our mind is the most important mechanism for providing control over our diet, exercise and all other aspects of our lives. The "picture" that we hold within our mind, is the "picture" of our life, and therefore it's our mind that determines our perspectives on everything, including what we eat, how much we eat, when we eat and more. Because of this, we'll return to some of this later in the book.

The "Calorie Counting" Diet Plans

Probably just like you, I've pretty much always been aware that eating foods containing a lot calories would cause weight gain. Accordingly, from time to time, I'd make an effort to keep track of the calories that I ate; I hoped that by doing this, I might be able to lose some weight. These attempts never really proved very successful; probably because I didn't really know much about how many calories I should be consuming, or even how to calculate any of that, in any meaningful fashion. Never the less, the concept seemed sound, but the way I was doing it just never seemed to work for me, at least not for very long.

I've never personally joined "Weight Watchers®", or any other similar organization that promotes weight loss. I'm certainly not against joining such organizations. I guess it's just that I'm not much of a "joiner", but I do understand the benefits of group dynamics, and I feel that for those who find comfort, and encouragement, in that setting, it seems to be a beneficial means for developing a solid dietary plan. Because I have never joined "Weight Watchers®", and not affiliated with "Weight Watchers®" in a way, I am hardly an expert on their program, or any of the other similar programs. I have, however, known a number of people who have participated in these programs, and they have been kind enough to share some of the broad concepts with me. To me, their basic concept of, "calories in - calories out", seems fundamentally sound.

Time and time again, I've read material by both physicians and dietitians that promoted the calorie counting concept for losing weight. The simple concept is that when your body takes in fewer calories than your body actually burns, you will lose weight. Of course, simple does not necessarily mean easy, and things rarely turn out to be that simple anyway. The whole thing seems to come down to having a fundamental understanding of how your body will physically react to the intake of fewer calories. There is, for example, always the possibility that your body could lose muscle mass, instead of fat, during the process, or you could encounter dizziness, and more. This is why most knowledgeable weight loss programs suggest that a person always consult with a physician, to be sure that any weight loss regiment is not personally detrimental. Most physicians will tell you that they were not subjected to very much dietary education in their original medical training, but many will also be very open to discussing your dietary ideas with you. This is something that I highly recommend for everyone to consider doing before going into any kind of serious diet regiment. I feel it's particularly important to listen to whether your physician feels that any specific dietary plan might be potentially harmful for you. If, of course, your physician has special dietary training, and/or is also a trained dietitian, their counsel on your dietary plans would likely be very useful.

Section III
Exercise and Weight Loss

Virtually every physician, dietician, as well as others seriously involved with weight loss say that engaging in regular light, or moderate, physical activity is beneficial. Yes we do need to get regular exercise, and as we begin to lose weight, we will naturally find that we want to increase our level of exercise. As we get thinner, exercise will become easier, and more enjoyable. There is, however, the caveat that exercise should not be overdone, and that the amount of exercise is different for each person; what's right for one person may not be right for the next. It's amazing that there are those with heart issues, and other serious health conditions, including those who are excessively obese, and those who are horribly out of shape, that fail to understand that they must use caution when exercising. All of us, and especially those with health issues, should seek professional medical advice prior to engaging in any new rigorous physical activity. The fact is that if you're healthy now, then engaging in regular light, or moderate, exercise is very likely good for you. But, adding new physical activates should always be done cautiously and sensibly, as you successfully progress down your weight loss path.

This book, however, is about weight loss, not about exercising or about physical fitness per se, so please don't think that I'm downplaying the importance of engaging in a program of regular exercise. An interesting book, one well worth reading, is "The Compound Effect" by Darren Hardy. The book starts with the fable of "The Tortoise and The Hare", to illustrate that it's those who stay in the race until the very end, that become the winners, and that those who sprint, and "crash" are simply out of the race. To me, that illustrates the most sensible way for starting a new weight loss, and/or exercise, regiment. As long as you're now getting a reasonable amount of exercise, it's my view that you should continue with your current level of physical activities. Before starting to add any significant new physical activities, you should focus on getting your weight loss program moving forward successfully.

Of course, if your current lifestyle is sedentary, and you don't regularly get some sort of regular exercise, after checking with a medical professional, you should probably start getting some sort of regular light physical activity. I do feel, however, that it can be counter productive to start too quickly with a burdensome, or aggressive, exercise program, as I believe that getting successfully started on the dietary portion of your weight loss program is your first priority, and is what makes the most practical sense. If you start with an exercise program that's too aggressive, you then run the risk of giving up not only on your exercise, but having that frustration spill over onto your entire weight loss program, and cause your entire effort to "crash". This is all about building a long-term successful weight loss program, so ease into developing a balanced weight loss plan, and allow the simple principles of doing, "one thing at a time", and "first things first", become your approach. Some people may disagree with this concept, but that's my view.

My feeling is that your exercise should be enjoyable for you, simply because enjoyable exercise is really the only kind of exercise capable of sustaining itself for the long-term, and creating the desired end result of making a you feel better, and becoming more productive. So why not start with some regular light exercise of any kind that you find enjoyable, an exercise that you know you can sustain. Once you've comfortably done that, and as your weight starts to drop, you'll want to start to slowly expand your exercise program, while still keeping it well within the limits of your personal physical ability. I find it unfortunate that there are people who put the primary focus on exercise for the purpose of weight loss, rather than first developing an effective weight loss eating regiment. It may be fine for those who are reasonably physically fit, to start with a full-fledged exercise program, but for many it's just not a good workable plan.

The fact of the matter is, for many people it's just plain physically and/or emotionally uncomfortable to exercise, perhaps because of age, being overweight, being totally out of shape, having joint pain and more. For this group especially, starting to exercise aggressively can be painful, and/or emotionally discouraging. When this happens along with the "stress" of a new dietary plan, the end result can too easily be the collapse of the entire weight loss plan.

To those who suggest that exercise should be the primary ingredient for a weight loss program, I don't want to say that's impossible, but I will point out that it does take a considerable amount of exercise to burn off excess fat. It's commonly understood that it requires about 3500 calories burned through exercise, for each pound of fat lost. To put that into context, to burn off 1 pound of fat, a typical person weighing 185 pounds would have to walk at 3 mph for over 11 hours, or play golf for almost 9 hours (about 36 holes), or run at 6 mph for almost 4 hours. Of course, these numbers are simply a rough guideline, and vary depending upon a number of conditions (especially the individuals weight), but it shows a fairly clear picture that exercise is only part of the weight loss picture.

Another important point to recognize is that although weight loss may not be easily achieved by just burning calories through exercise, the addition of exercise to a proper diet, does have a positive affect on your body's ability to efficiently burn calories. This synergism between making positive dietary changes, and exercise, is why it's so important to have at least some sustainable exercise occurring, right from the start of you weight loss program.

Now, I know that there are those who will say, *"no pain, no gain"*, and for some things I'm in that camp too. But the cold hard fact of life is that we all tend to do what we "want" to do, and doing things that are painful, or emotionally uncomfortable, is a very fast way to find discouragement, and quickly turn the entire effort into something that we simply don't to do at all. Most of us have long ago learned that the starting of any difficult task is by far the hardest part of the entire task. If you want your weight loss program to work effectively, then it's important to start with a well-balanced plan that will work for you, and will keep on working. You'll find that changing your eating habits, and your caloric intake, will not be a particularly easy task in itself, so please don't add too much to your plan, too soon; take your time, just like the "tortoise", that's you're best chance to win this race.

As a final thought on exercise, I offer a quote from something that President Richard Nixon once said in jest to a reporter, but which I feel also contains a great deal of wisdom. President Nixon said, *"The best exercise that I know of for losing weight, is to push yourself away from the dinner table"*.

Section IV
Obstacles That Lie Ahead

We all realize that weight loss isn't easy, so let's talk a little bit about the weight related obstacles that we're likely to face. We need to be able to recognize, and anticipate, what roadblocks we're likely to encounter, and more importantly what we need do to avoid them. Every one of us is going to have to deal with our obstacles, those things that seem to try to block our weight loss path. Overcoming these obstacles is a major key to our achieving a successful, and healthy, weight loss/maintenance program.

Although there has been much written on the subject of basic human instincts, at the top of the list is the basic instinct for survival, for which food is at the top of the survival list. The reason that I bring this up is simply to illustrate that the human desire for food is absolutely natural. What is perhaps less than natural is the habit of excessively eating more food than is necessary for our survival. In short, excessive overeating is simply not a natural behavior. Some will point out that the building up of fat is an instinct for survival to help carry us through both famine, and cold winters. This may well be true, but in our society today, I believe that our excessive overeating is a learned behavior, and is clearly an obstacle that we must all overcome.

As a result of the structured lifestyle that we live, there are other obstacles that get in the way of our maintaining a stable healthy weight. For example, we're all pretty much trained to have breakfast, lunch and dinner, as our major sources for food. We tend to do this is in spite of the fact that we may, or may not, be hungry at the time, or whether we may, or may not, actually need the food. On top of that, typically breakfast is our smallest meal, lunch is a medium-size meal and dinner (supper) is the largest meal, which is probably backwards from the way it should be. The long and the short of this is that we tend to eat three structured meals, when perhaps fewer meals, or maybe even more meals, might actually be better for us. We also tend to eat the meals in sizes configured by society, rather than by our own personal needs. For example, restaurants long ago learned that it was profitable to raise the portion size of meals, as they could then justify higher prices by making us feel like we were getting a special value. More importantly, restaurants were now able to attract the all-important customer that has become accustomed to the new norm of overeating. With restaurants serving these large portions, customers could now easily justify (in their mind) eating the entire large food portion, simply because the restaurant served it to them; the reasoning being, "after all, everyone is doing it".

As restaurant customers, there are lots of games that we play. We tell ourselves, that going to the restaurant is a celebration, and therefore it's okay to overeat the large quantities of food that's served. And, when we go to a buffet we tell ourselves that since it's a bargain, it's okay for us to go back and get multiple food refills. It's all really a game that we play, just so that we can satisfy our "want" for the satisfaction of good tasting food. The businessperson, and their clients, going out to dinner on expense accounts tell themselves that this is business, so let's all celebrate by ordering large portions of rich food. Of course, there are many more food games than these; I'm sure that you know some, and that when you stop and think about it, you'll uncover a few games of your own.

The reality is that most of us simply like to eat more than we should because we find eating very satisfying, and enjoyable. Additionally, when some of us become stressed, the satisfaction of eating seemingly becomes an effective way to make us feel good, and relieve our stressful feelings. Because we are all so different, and the human mind is so powerful, there is literally a limitless number of different ways for us to convince ourselves that it's okay to be eating whatever it is that we "want", as much as we "want", and whenever we "want". It is impossible here, to try to define every individual disguise used to indulge all of our personal food habits.

Understanding the Enemy

Other obstacles lie ahead; I like to think of them as the enemy. Do you have any idea as to which foods people find most attractive? Perhaps you are not aware of it, but long ago restaurants figured out that foods containing sugar, salt and fats were the foods that were the most food attractive to their customers. Let's be clear about this, the sole purpose of any business is to make a profit (otherwise it would be called a charity), and because restaurants are profit-making businesses, they're more concerned about selling their food, than whether or not their meals are sized properly, or nutritionally sound for their customers. Simply put, the food flavors of salt, sugar and fat, are very effective in satisfying the desires of restaurant customers, and are therefore good for the restaurant business. For many years the public failed to realize why the french fries in some restaurants tasted so much better than others. It was because they not only had the flavor of salt, and fat, but sugar was also added. It was only a few years ago that a number of restaurants were virtually forced to remove the added sugar from their french fry products.

I like to use the phrase that "sugar is the enemy", but that's simply to remind me that eating simple sugars does nothing much for me, other than to create fat. Most people understand this concept fairly clearly, but many fail to understand that simple carbohydrates, those like potatoes, bread and pasta, are converted into fat in same manner as sugar. To make matters worse, most of those simple starchy foods are normally eaten in conjunction with butter, cheesy sauces and sugar filled condiments, all of which join together to become the enemy of those trying to manage their weight.

Personally, you could say that I'm blessed by the fact that sweets are not an overly important flavor to me. On the other hand, my downfall is that I really enjoy the taste of fatty foods. I would choose a hamburger over a piece of cake, pie or candy, every time. The point is we are all different, and we all have our own set of "food enemies", and it is up to each of us to spend the time, and effort, to identify them, and learn how to modify our eating habits so as to reduce those fattening foods that we truly "want" to eat, but don't really need.

Celebrations

Another obstacle that I want to mention is the social norms of using food to celebrate. Most of us have lives that are filled with customs, and traditions, that revolve around food. Virtually every holiday is a cause for people to gather together and celebrate, almost always including food. It could be the hotdogs on the Fourth of July, the turkey and dressing at Thanksgiving, the ham, desserts and other tasty trimmings of the holiday seasons, there are the romantic dinners for Valentines, the festive parties for St. Patrick's Day and more. As if the holidays weren't enough there are the ever-present birthdays, weddings and other celebrations, both at work and at home. The tradition of overeating at these occasions has become the norm, and it becomes another huge obstacle for us to overcome, while we're working hard to sustain our weight loss program.

"Cop-Outs" That We Hear And Use

"Cop-Outs" are obstacles with which I'm sure we're all familiar. "Cop-Outs" are the excuses that are so prevalent in our society today. It's bad enough that there will be some people, well-meaning or not, who are essentially working against our weight loss success, but when we join with them by our using a "cop-out", we start working against ourselves too, and we become doomed to failure virtually before we start. Let's take a look at the kinds of things that we sometimes hear others saying, and which are things that we might hear ourselves saying, too.

"I don't want to be skinny, I'm happy just the way I am", "You're not fat, you're just healthy", "Being heavy, runs in my family", "I am just a big-boned person", "My energy level drops off, and I need to eat something with sugar in it right now", "I can't lose weight because I have a medical condition", "Society just wants us to be skinny so they can sell us more clothing, but I'm happy just the way I am", "I'm happy with my weight, you'll just have to accept me the way I am", and, "I just naturally have a slow metabolism, and there's nothing I can do about that".

Let's be clear about ourselves, and our individual metabolic rates, which simplistically is the rate at which our bodies consume, or utilize, energy. Contrary to what some people think, metabolic rates differs only slightly from person to person. In some cases it's possible that this kind of difference could be hereditary, but with that said, some studies have shown that these differences typically vary less than 8% between most individuals. Other studies also show that metabolic rates are likely to drop by about 5% after age forty. So even if an individual used 2000 calories a day, and in my opinion that's a lot, a 10% difference would mean that one person might utilize 200 calories a day, more or less than another person. To put that into perspective, 200 calories is roughly equal to 2 tablespoons of peanut butter, or about a half of a large cheeseburger (no fries), and who among us can't adjust for that small difference if we choose to? Like it or not, metabolism wise, we are all about the same; and for almost all us, the fact is that our being overweight is simply the result of a lot of small personal eating choices that we've made over time.

The "cop-out" excuses shown above, and many more like them, are just excuses created either by ourselves, or by others. The only reason that all of these excuses exist is to try to make us feel better about our over-weight condition; yes we're trying to kid ourselves. These excuses are all just an attempt to create an artificial comfort-level for us, even though we know that we are heavier then we should be for our own well-being. If we're going to succeed on our path to weight loss success, we simply must stop being a party to the "cop-outs" like these, and when we hear them, we must stop ourselves in our tracks, and not be tempted to use them. These comments can serve no useful purpose in our future weight loss efforts.

This section of the book was to illustrate some of the many obstacles faced by all of us when dealing with weight loss. It's important that we identify, and understand, our enemies, if we are to defeat them. These obstacles are our enemies, and they will stand in our way until we develop our own individual ways to eliminate them.

Section V
Why The Path Is Difficult

You'll see that as we move onto other sections of this book, the path to successful weight loss is relatively simple, but unfortunately simple does not mean easy, or painless. Achieving successful long-term weight loss can be difficult, especially if we decide to let it be difficult. Almost every difficulty that we'll encounter on this road to weight loss, will be self-imposed. In this section we'll look at some of the most common ways that we try to make all of this difficult for ourselves.

Fear Of Failure

A basic truth of life is that we must all deal with ourselves, and the demons in our own minds. Many of us are conditioned to think that failure is bad, and because of that, we fear failure. Actually, if you think about it seriously, many of the key lessons that we've learned in life, were learned as the result of some kind of failure, or mistake, that we made. It's really hard to learn from success, as it's quite often unclear what specifically may have gone so right as to caused the success. But, when things go wrong, it's usually pretty clear just where the problem lies, making it easy to make adjustments toward a better course the next time. Everyone experiences numerous failures in their life; failure is a normal human experience, but some people will lament in failure, while others relish the opportunity to move ahead on a better course. The trick, of course, is to try to keep your failures small, and your successes big. So, please don't fear failure, it's a natural part of everyone's life, and natural learning process.

I think it useful to be aware of the importance of the lessons that are learned from failure. For example, I'm willing to bet that you've failed on other diets before, maybe many. I know that if you allow the fear of failure to plague you right from the start, you'll be starting this project with "one arm behind your back". So please enter this project, and "fear not", you'll encounter some set backs, and you'll have weeks where you struggle, and you may actually gain a pound or two, but so what, just learn from it, and move forward. Fear is simply a thought in your mind, so just replace that thought with the positive thoughts of your weight loss success, and keep moving forward.

Friends and Relatives

If our path to weight loss success weren't difficult, then losing weight wouldn't be such a huge problem for us either. If we only had to deal with designing a diet, as some would have you believe, then things would be a whole lot easier.

Let's look at the weight loss quagmire that we all face. And, right off the bat, we have to deal with our friends, relatives and often coworkers. Most are well meaning, and encouraging, but you still end up hearing things like, "just this once, forget your diet, and enjoy a taste of some wonderful food". Then there are those who are envious, or jealous, of your weight loss progress, and may even make hurtful remarks to try to undermine your progress. Each of us is different, and each of us must find our own way to handle these situations individually, so let's look a few possible situations, and what you might want to do.

The well-meaning comment, that doesn't come out quite right: example: "Wow, you've lost a lot of weight, but I always thought that you looked good at your old weight". Your answer: Just smile, and say, "Thank you", and nothing more. Don't allow yourself to engage in any conversation that causes you to defend your weight loss program, or how you may (or may not) have looked before you started. It's probably best to just politely walk away from this conversation.

The well-meaning comment that comes out right: example: "You're looking great". Just smile and say "Thank you", but no need to walk away this time, you just got a nice compliment, and this is obviously a supportive friend.

The nasty, or envious, comment, an example: "I'm glad that you're finally doing something about your weight". Or, "I really don't know why you're putting yourself through all of that, you looked just fine before". Just politely say, "Thank you, I'm feeling really good about my progress", then turn and walk away; don't allow yourself to be drawn into a conversation about any aspect of your weight loss program, these people may be "friends", but they are not necessarily being supportive.

The bottom line is that you've engaged in this weight loss program for yourself, not for other people. It is rude, and impolite, for others to try to drag you into conversations about your weight loss program, it's your program, not theirs. So, share it with your true friends if you like, but never feel obligated to do so, and never allow yourself to get involved in a defensive, or negative conversation about weight loss. Success is already on your side, so just keep it there.

Your Habits and Training

What kind of "bad" eating habits do you have? We all have them, and they're a really big part of our problem with weight. Of course we're going to have to do something about these habits, but before we can do that, we need to identify as many of these "bad" habits that we can. Here's a list of many of the obvious poor eating habits, but there are plenty more of them, too.

Eating Too Fast: It takes time for your stomach to react to the food that you eat, and start giving you a feeling of being full. When you eat too fast, you almost always end up eating too much before your body starts to tell you that you're full.

Continual Snacking: Another name for this is "emotional eating", or eating out habit or "feel good" eating, all of which occur mostly because you've kept the most wonderful treats conveniently located where they're easy for you find, and get to. Eliminate treats from your house, or at least locate them somewhere inconvenient for you.

Taking Second (And Third) Helpings: This is mostly eating out of habit, along with the availability of extra food, not because your body needs the food. Cook only the amount of food you need for your meal, you'll be much better off.

Drinking Regular (Sugar) Soda Pop: There is absolutely no reason that someone interested in losing weight should consume this beverage. Regular (sugar) soda pop takes a direct route to becoming the newest fat in your body. There are lots of alternatives to drinking this beverage, and to say that you drink it because you don't like the taste of anything else, simply indicates that you've become dependant (addicted) to the taste of sugar, and that's a weight loss nightmare.

Adding Cheese To The Things You Eat: Almost everyone loves cheese, but cheese is a fat product that contains a lot of calories. You don't have to avoid all cheese, but adding it to burgers, to eggs, to vegetables and etc., simply masks the original taste of the main food with a cheese flavor, and most importantly adds a lot of extra calories.

Eating Out, When You Can Eat At Home: Eating at a restaurant, especially a "fast-food" restaurant, almost always invites you to over-eat, calorie wise; very few "fast food" restaurants are weight-loss friendly.

Eating Everything On Your Plate: Perhaps when you were young, you were told to eat everything that was put on your plate. I have no interest in getting into whether or not that's a good practice of not, it makes absolutely no difference now. You're grown, and there is no one telling you to eat everything that's on your plate, so just stop eating when you're no longer hungry.

Drinking Beer Or Alcoholic Beverages In Excess: It's not necessary to cut out all alcoholic beverages to be on a weight loss diet, in fact if they are part of your normal life (and you're healthy), then a diet without any, might not easily sustain itself. On the other hand, alcohol converts to calories in your body, and those beverages that contain sugar in addition to the alcohol, simply have even more calories. Know your beverages, and their calories, and if you choose to drink these kinds of beverages, then drink them in moderation.

Relying Too Much On Frozen/Prepared Meals: There is nothing intrinsically wrong with many of the frozen meals, in fact "Weight Watchers®", and others, have some fine lower calorie meals that may be worth investigating. The issues with many of the prepared frozen meals are that they are loaded with starch, sugar and cheese. In addition, with many brands the containers play the calorie verses serving size game, where the container gives a serving size that's really only a small portion of a realistic serving size. However, the real problem occurs when we regularly rely on these prepared meals for a quick meal, when we'd be much better off to take a few more minutes and prepare a fresh healthy meal, with lean meat and vegetables.

Snacking On Chips and Dip: We're talking straight calories here, no significant nutritional value, and it's just "fun to eat" food. It's best to avoid these altogether, and find a low-calorie substitute snack that better fits your weight loss program.

I'll bet that you've identified with some of these bad habits; well, so did I. The fact is if we're serious about losing weight, we're going to have to address our bad habits, and more. So start making a list now, of all the habits that you're going to need to change; we'll be addressing how to do that later in this book.

The Food Police

Of course, there's actually no food police, but then again there should be, and you'd be wise to appoint yourself to a life term in that position. I'm sorry, but it's your job to see to it that the wonderful fattening foods that you love to over-eat so much are removed from your pantry and refrigerator. The temptation created by all of the great tasting treats that you've been kept conveniently located in the past, is simply too great. If you choose to continue to keep these foods around, it will make your weight loss journey much more difficult. I'm not suggesting that the your new diet can't contain these foods; it should allow some of treats that you love, but with controlled moderation. You know what these foods are, they're your personal favorites, so now is the time to start being accountable, and become your own personal food police. So, don't keep an extra amount of your favorite fattening foods, just sitting around where they're easy for you to snack on. This change alone will be a huge help in making your weight loss program successful.

Your Clothes

One of the issues that we all face in losing weight is that as we lose weight, our clothes get loose and unflattering. Of course, if you have a history of "yo-yo" dieting, you may still have a few smaller sizes around, and needless to say if money's not an object, then none of this applies to you. For the rest of us, it can be an issue because we're reluctant to buy new wardrobes that may also soon be too large. On the other hand, we work so hard to achieve our weight loss that the last thing we want to start doing is to look "dumpy", or unstylish, during the process. So, here are a few suggestions.

Don't buy a whole new wardrobe until you have reached your target weight, but occasionally treat yourself to something new, stylish and that accents your new weight loss. Also, there are many clothing styles that are flexible, and can fit nicely over a range of sizes.

Look to your good friends, or family from whom you may be able to borrow, or trade, a few appropriate garments, it can augment your few new ones.

Alter the nice garments that you have, there may not be a tailor shop on every corner anymore, but most laundries have that service, or have someone that they can recommend.

Almost every community has some "lightly used" designer clothing stores where you can find some very nice garments, at reasonable prices. Many of these stores take clothes in on consignment, so just maybe you can offset some of the cost of some new interim clothes, by selling your larger size clothes through the same consignment store.

These are just a few suggestions, be creative and find a way to keep looking your best as you lose weight. When you're proud of how you look, you feel better, you're more upbeat and positive, and that's very important, as it's a critical part of maintaining your weight loss enthusiasm.

Section VI
Why Change Is Necessary

This book is about losing weight, and keeping it off, as well as how to make the life changes necessary to accomplish that task; the book is not intended to explore the many other important related issues. There are other issues that you may wish to explore independently, such as nutrition, food additives, exercise routines, and general health matters all of which are important in their own right. But, I would be remiss if I didn't touch on one very important health related subject, simply because it relates directly to why losing weight should be important to all of us.

The Associated Press-NORC Center for Public Affairs Research recently conducted a national household survey, to measure (among other things) the general public's opinions about obesity-related health issues in the United States. The survey showed that the public had a clear understanding that obesity can damage your health, and openly acknowledged that excessive weight would likely accelerate the risk for both heart attack and diabetes. But, the public showed very little awareness that carrying excessive weight was also a likely contributing factor for many other diseases. That list includes cancer (colon, breast, prostrate, uterus and more), arthritis and joint pain, high blood pressure, high cholesterol, stroke, sleep apnea, depression, asthma, sexual dysfunction, infertility and more.

By pointing this out, I simply wish to illustrate that regardless of what your personal motivating issue is for losing weight, there are many other "built in" benefits for weight loss that may also accrue, so let's get back on track with the subject at hand.

This is the most important section of this entire book, because it's about the changes that you're going to want to make, if you're serious about long-term weight loss. Let's face it, with any weight loss plan, you're asking yourself to change your behavior away from a behavior that you're currently finding easy and enjoyable. Change is never pleasant, change is always uncomfortable, change isn't easy and frankly, nobody that I've ever met likes change at all; we all tend to resist change, it's a very natural reaction. With that said, the fact is that the more that you truly want to make a weight loss change in your life, the easier these changes will be.

Most of the information about weight loss seems to focus on the kinds of foods that we must eat, and the diet that we must be embrace. It's simply a shortsighted point of view to think that some pre-set diet plan, set by someone else, will be the long-term cure to our weight loss dilemma. The plain and simple truth is that food in itself does not cause of weight gain, it's our personal eating decisions that are the real cause. The only thing that any diet plan can do is to try to force us into eating, differently than the way that our mind has been telling us that we want to eat. Not one of us likes to be forced into doing something that we don't want to do. In the end, we really don't want to eat those special weight loss diets forever, and that's why they end up falling to the side, and we go back into the weight loss yo-yo club. It's not that those diet plans won't work, it's they can only work short term unless we find a way for our minds to fully embrace the fact that we want to be eating like that forever. The fact is that over our lifetime, our personal wants and desires will cause the actual foods we eat, and diet format we use, to naturally be in constant change. This means that any weight loss plan that will be effective long-term, must be driven by our wants and desires, not by some diet rules set forth by others.

It's our own individual mindset that we must change, our mind controls our behavior, and our behavior controls the things that we eat, as well as the exercise that we choose to get. That's why the primary thrust of this book is about the changes that we must make within ourselves, and how we can effectively make those changes in order to achieve the long-term weight loss that each of us desires.

This section is about how you can, and must, retrain your thinking, and do it in a way that's totally customized to fit your uniqueness, your desires, your situation and your personality. In fact that's the key; if you're asked to retrain your thinking to follow a plan that was created by someone else, it's pretty unlikely that you'll follow that plan for very long. That's why your program will be designed by you, and for you. After all, we all like our own ideas, so now's your chance to design your own food diet, one that you'll truly like because you created it with foods that you enjoy eating. You'll also be making changes in your own behavior, but again those changes will be designed and implemented by you. All of this will create a customized weight loss framework for you that you can easily embrace as your own, and which will start to feel both enjoyable, and comfortable. All of this will be much different than any weight loss experience that you've had in the past.

A Process For The Long Term

Mapping out your own unique, and customized, weight loss plan, including the changes you'll want to make in your behavior, can take anywhere from a few hours, to a few years, it's all going to be up to you. I will do my very best to guide you through the process for making these changes, but it must be you that actually designs, and implements your changes. The good news is that these changes will specifically fit your personality, and your personal situation. The rest of the good news is that you will actually start to enjoy your new dedicated commitment, concentration, and weight loss discipline. The bottom line turns out to be that it's not the new foods that you eat that creates weight loss, it's your food related behavior, including the new way that you begin to feel about food, that will change your weight, and life, forever.

In the rest of this section, we will discuss some changes needed in order for you to achieve your desired weight, and to sustain it on a long-term basis. After you've completely read this book, and taken some time to fully digest all of its information, I feel that you'll see how simple this process actually is, and how achievable it will be for you. I continually refer to long-term weight loss, and there's a reason for that. Short-term weight loss is relatively easy to achieve by simply making a short term forced reduction in what you eat, but that kind of uncomfortable change will be not be sustainable for the long term, once you return to your old established comfortable eating habits. The weight is lost, and then it returns again, and now you're back into the "yo-yo" club. This book is about long-term, life-changing, weight loss, and that's going to require permanent changes in your life. The concepts that I will introduce to you, are ones that I bring from the business world, where I, as well as others, have been successfully able to use them in business. Using this kind of approach is the only successful way that I've ever seen, for making permanent behavioral changes, and I know that they can work for you too. There is an organized process for making these kinds of changes, and I will do my best to explain exactly how you can tackle the process, each step along the way. Please don't get discouraged, as what you will learn may help you with making many other positive changes in your life, too.

Ground Rules

The basic rule for everyone, before starting a weight loss or exercise plan, is to first seek the advice of a physician, or medical professional, to be sure that you're healthy enough to make an exercise, and/or dietary change, in your life.

The next rule is that this is not a race, it's not about the first one to get to the weight loss finish line; it's about the one who gets to the finish line and then stays at the finish line. This is all about taking one small step at a time, and then to just keep taking step, after step, after step, after step. Weight loss with slow steady long-term progress is what you want, and it's that slow progress that will stay with you for the long haul. The math is simple, if you lose one ounce a day, for the next year, you will have lost over 22 pounds, with minimal sacrifice. The instant gratification world that we live in today, allows us to easily believe that everything should happen quickly, but unfortunately that's not the way it is in "real life". I'll remind you again about the children's story of "The Tortoise, and The Hare"; that old fable is a very real example of the program on which you're about to embark.

Along the same line, this next rule is that you must "keep your eye on the ball". As every successful athlete will tell you, you must have steadfast focus on the target that's immediately in front of you. The football player makes a touchdown not by watching the goal line, but by watching the spinning pass as it comes into his hands, and it's then that he finds the goal line. The baseball player doesn't look out to the fence where he wants his ball to go, his focus is on acutely watching the ball in that micro-second that his bat hits the ball, and it's only after seeing the ball hit the bat, that the thought of hitting it over the fence, might occur. And so it is with your diet plan, your focus must always stay with what's happening in the moment, you must keep your focus on the food that's in front of you, and on the eating decisions you make while you're eating.

Another rule, as basic as it may be, is that you must be willing to take responsibility. There is no other way to do any of this without your willingness to be totally and fully responsible for your mindset, your decisions and for your actions. That means that there will be reasons for things occasionally not going as planned, but that there's never an excuse, there's no blaming other people, and there's no blaming outside circumstances. Responsibility means accountability, it means that you're the one who's fully in charge of yourself, and it's you who must be accountable for yourself, and for all of the results that you desire to achieve. To many this may sound harsh, but it's a reality of life, and it must be an absolute reality for your weight loss effort, if you're to achieve the long-term weight loss that you desire.

The final ground rule is that you must keep this process enjoyable, maybe even find a way to make it fun, like perhaps giving yourself rewards along the way. This is not to downplay that many of the changes that you'll be making will initially be difficult, and perhaps uncomfortable. The fact is that in the beginning, some of the dietary changes that you decide to make may not be as comfortable for you as was your previous diet. The truth is that if you don't keep this process enjoyable for you, there's a great likelihood that you may abandon it altogether. Because of this, it's important that the changes you set for yourself stay within reasonable bounds, and that the dietary changes that you choose to make continue to include some of the same foods that you now enjoy, though likely in smaller quantities.

Learning The Secret

These next couple paragraphs may seem confusing at first, as the subject of "wanting" something, versus "needing" something, can be difficult to understand. The difference is that a "want" is a voluntary choice, and a "need" is something that's originates involuntarily, outside of our personal control.

For example, we clearly "need" nutrition in order to sustain life, so that's a "need"; clearly we didn't choose that voluntarily. If only one food possibility exists in the face of starvation, then there's no choice to be made, as survival is a basic instinct. But, when there are multiple food choices, we can then make a decision, which creates a "want"; and, it's now something for which we are accountable.

My point here is that we don't necessarily "need" to eat indulgent foods, or to eat in excess just to survive; those are food choices that we make simply because that's what we "want", or desire. And, in making our choice, we also become accountable for the choices of what we eat, as it's clearly not a case of survival. So, the real question becomes, why would we make choices that work against us, by choosing to eat foods that clearly work against our weight loss, when we also know that we "want" to lose weight, too.

Paradoxical choices like this occur because there's a reason "why" that stands behind every choice that we're faced with, and the "why" that stands behind one of those choices is simply stronger, and more motivational, than the "why" behind the other choice. For example, let's say that you're someone who loves to eat rich fast food, and your reason "why" is because it really tastes great to you, plus it's a quick, convenient and easy way to eat. Now, you know that eating too much food like that will work against your weight loss, but you eat the fast food anyway. Here's the key to all of this, the reason "why" you eat the fast food, is simply because (in this example) your "why" of wanting the food that tastes great, is stronger than the reason "why" you want to lose weight; seriously, it's that simple. I guarantee that the reason that one "why" is stronger than the other is rooted somewhere deep within your inner "feelings", it's not simply a conscience, or "thinking", choice.

The secret to weight loss victory lies in your ability to fully embrace your weight loss "why". You must allow your "why" to be strong enough to successfully guide you safely past the choices of the many great tasting foods that will reach out to you during your weight loss journey. But, making the choice to harness this secret is 100% up to you. You're acceptance of this one simple point, will allow you to experience the power of your weight loss "why", and you'll begin to feel it motivate you toward the achievement of your weight loss victory.

I find it interesting that we all seem to instantly know what it is that we "want", and then our brain instantly finds ingenious ways to rationalize those choices; and, do it in a ways that allow us to believe that we are actually filling a "need", rather than acting on a "want". We are all individually accountable for everything that we want, but we often kid ourselves into believing that those things are a "need", and that's probably because we automatically know that our needs are situational, and involuntary, so therefore they're not something for which we're personally accountable. Needless to say, this is all simply a mind game to avoid accountability for the choices we make, and of course we're the only people who are getting fooled.

An example of disguising a want for a need, might be a person who says they are starving, simply because it's lunchtime and their stomach may be growling. That individual might even say something like, "I'm starving, and I need to get something to eat before I pass out". We all know deep down that it's highly unlikely that person is going to pass out, unless of course they have a serious medical issue, in which case it should be attended to accordingly. What they're really saying is that their stomach is growling, which is likely occurring because they've created the habit of eating at this same time every day. A growling stomach can be slightly annoying, and perhaps even a little uncomfortable, so they've convinced themselves that their body actually "needs" the food, when a glass of water might quiet the growling stomach just as well. What they're really doing is kidding themselves into believing that they have a "need" for food, rather than being accountable for the fact that they simply "want" the food.

From this example, we can start to see how easily we can attempt to justify our desire to eat as a "need" to eat, but if you've ever said to yourself that you felt guilty for indulging in some excess food, then you've just felt your weight loss "why", reaching out in an instinctive effort to make you feel accountable. And, when you learn to strengthen your weight loss "why" so that it gives you the support you need before you indulge, you'll be well on your way to achieving the weight loss you so desire.

What's Your Secret?

We've just talked a little about your weight loss "why", but if you're not familiar with the concept, it may still seem a little foggy, but I assure you that it's very important. The simple concept of learning to deeply understand "why" you truly want to lose weight is the very heart of this entire weight loss process. I know that sounds strangely simple, but it's actually much more involved than it sounds. No matter what it is in life that you decide to do, you choose to do it because you want to do it, and behind your "wants", there are your personal reasons "why" you want to do it, and it's those "whys" that actually drive you to do all of the things that you choose to do.

Stop and think about that for a minute; anything and everything that we choose to do in life, has a very personal "why" buried somewhere behind it, and, it's that "why" that keeps us on course to the completion of our chosen tasks. And, it will be your weight loss "why" that will keep you from drifting off your path to weight loss success. The truth is that your weight loss "why" will be the most powerful long-term force for consistency, and stability, for your weight loss journey.

If asked, your first reaction might be to say something like "the reason why I want to lose weight is because I want look better, feel better and have more energy". But, is that truly your deep-seated personal "why"? It might be, but I suspect not. I suspect that there's a much deeper, and more specific, "why" that's really driving your desire for weight loss. Perhaps being thinner will help you find a romantic match, or perhaps allow you to perform better at a certain sport, maybe it's a specific personal health issue, or an emotional need, and there's an awful lot of other very real possibilities. Your "why" is something that's very personal to you, and to you alone; it's your own, very powerful weight loss secret motivation! It takes a considerable amount of personal soul searching, to get to your true deep-seated "why". One of the reasons it's so difficult, is that the root source for your "why" is always generated through your "feelings", not through your "thinking". For whatever reason, many people have a very difficult time getting in touch with their true feelings, most likely their "thinking" tends to get in their way, which makes the search for their true weight loss "why" that much more difficult. Again, your "why" is not created through logical thought, it is created from your deepest personal inner feelings.

The root of your deep-seated weight loss "why", is likely some very sensitive personal feelings as to how you actually want to feel, or see yourself, when you become a thin person. Perhaps that sounds confusing, but think about that for a minute, and let it sink in, as it's your key to clearing the path to successful weight loss and weight maintenance. Our human systems seem to automatically guide us to choose those things that we "want", and beneath those choices lays our true inner feelings of "why" we want those things, and this is the core force that we seek to identify. In the simplest terms, if eating food gives you a better feeling than the feeling you get by seeing yourself as a thin person, you're going to eat food to just to feel good, rather than to eat the foods that will aid your weight loss. Conversely, if you have an inner view of yourself as a thin person, and the feeling that gives you is more wonderful than anything you've ever felt before in your life, you'll just as naturally eat only when your body needs the food, because you see yourself feeling better as a thin person, than you do as a person that indulges in food just to feel good in the moment.

Unfortunately, our "why" lies much deeper than our conscience level of thinking; our "why" lies nestled within our deepest emotions and feelings. It's one thing to accept something logically, and yet another thing to completely embrace it as our own personal feeling. An

42

example that most people quickly understand is the feeling of love; when you think about it, it's basically impossible to think yourself into being in love, love is something that you must feel deep down. And, so it is with your future thinness. Trying to think your way there simply doesn't work, but once you can actually feel yourself as being thin, believing within your mind that you are thin, then you're well on your way. Simply stated, you must fall in love with your thin self, before you can become your thin self that you love. And, when you begin to create a deep belief within yourself that you truly love the feeling of being your new thin self, you will start to instinctively feel that being thin, feels much better than the feeling you get from eating food, just because it tastes good.

What makes us feel good about weight loss is not always immediately obvious, in fact identifying our true feelings about becoming a thin person, can be a very illusive and difficult. On the surface, we might simply say that being thin will make us feel good, because we'll have more energy, have the ability to wear more stylish clothes, or because it will make us more popular. The truth may be that we truly have a deep desire to be thin, but the truth may also be that over time we have convinced ourselves that we feel quite a bit differently about our weight situation, and about ourselves. If that sounds complicated it's because it is, our mind is a very complicated place.

It's impossible for others, no matter who they may be, to tell us how we feel! Our deepest feelings and desires are almost always one thing, while what we choose to share with others, and what we tell our sub-conscience mind, can often be something much different. Our sub-conscience mind is non-judgmental, and when we fill it with "garbage thoughts", namely all the nonsense that we've fed it about indulgent foods, poor eating habits and more, our mind can be completely unaware of our true inner feelings and desires. Even when our deepest desires may truly be for weight loss, our mind only knows to produce a "why" based on the "garbage thoughts" its been fed.

In the end, everything we do is derived from those thoughts within our mind, and eventually any "why" brought on by "garbage thoughts", will drive our actions toward the achievement of that same "garbage". Conversely, when our mind is fed good positive weight loss thoughts generated from our deepest inner feelings and desires, no matter how secret those feelings may be, we will then start to be driven by a new, and very positive weight loss "why". In other words, if the thoughts we've pushed into our mind makes us feel better about indulgent eating, than it makes us feel about being thin, then it's indulgent eating that we'll keep doing.

It's taken some of us many years to reach the weight that we are today, and every step along the way we've silently talked to ourselves, and given ourselves all kinds of "garbage" reasons for why it was okay to be our current weight. The silent self-talk, whether it be the excuse we give ourselves for buying sweets, for taking second helpings of food, or for buying larger sized clothes, it all gets recorded in our sub-conscience mind, and all of those self-talk conversations become the basis for the "why" that drives our eating. Like the computer wizards always say, "garbage in, garbage out", so as long as you're feeding your mind with thoughts that let you feel that your current weight is okay, then any weight loss effort you attempt to make, is undermined from the very start.

Learning to feel good about weight loss, and about your future thin self is not necessarily easily done. For example, if you feel that your being thin might cause you to be the center of attention, and if you felt that being the center of attention would make you uncomfortable, then you're naturally going to have an automatic feeling that losing weight isn't beneficial to you, which in turn might even allow you to feel good about indulgent eating. Unfortunately, that kind of thinking could actually end up creating a feeling that being heaver makes you feel more comfortable, secure and happy, than being thin.

You may say "nonsense", of course being thin would make me happy, but the truth is that this is between you, and your inner self, your feelings can't be right or wrong, they're simply your feelings, you own them and you control them. No one else can change your feelings; you're the person that's 100% responsible for your feelings. Of course, the above example is only an illustration of how complex the concept of feeling good about weight loss can actually be. This simply points out that at some point, we're all going to have to "get in touch" with our true feelings about weight loss. And, at that point we'll need to start to create new thoughts that will support our successful weight loss, (we'll discuss how we can do this in a following section). It's only when we can achieve this deep feeling of happiness about being a thin person that we can successfully start down the path to weight loss success.

The bottom line is that before we can successfully maintain long-term weight loss, we must first internalize deep within our mind that the end result of our weight loss will truly make us feel wonderful. And, until we've done the soul-searching necessary to fully understand "why" being a thinner person will make us feel wonderful, we are destined to continue a life of yo-yo weight loss, at best. Conversely, as soon as we start to grasp the deep reason "why" our losing weight will create an exhilarating and happy feeling for us, we will have true clarity as to "why" weight loss is so very important to us, and that in turn will drive us on a successful weight loss journey.

Unlocking The Secret

To start the process of finding your weight loss "why", just sit back, relax and let your mind just drift with your feelings; the more you do this, the easier it will become, and the more progress that you'll start to make. You might even try taking a deep breath, and then exhaling it quickly. Do this a few times, but take your time and don't rush between deep breaths, this may well help you to "let go", and to relax.

Finding your deep-seated weight loss "why", may take you days, weeks, months, or even longer, as this is a journey that must be taken one step at a time. But, it's a journey that's well worth the effort, as your future thinness is dependant on the truth, and strength, of your weight loss "why".

When you begin to discover your "why", you will find that it will need to be strengthened and supported, so we'll cover how you can do that, in a section that follows. But, when you're confident that you've found your true "why", and you begin to allow it to sink deeply into your subconscious mind, your purpose will become crystal clear, and your motivation and enthusiasm for keeping steadfastly on your path to your weight loss success, will begin to soar.

I assure you that the identification of your deep-seated weight loss "why" is critical to the success of your weight loss program. If you have even the slightest doubt about that, I encourage you to learn more on this very important subject. I personally like the excellent book, "Start With Why", by Simon Sinek. There is also a very informative YouTube online video of Simon Sinek delivering a short talk on the importance of "why", I recommend that you Google "TED video, Start With Why", and you should find it easily, it's very much worth watching.

If you are serious about achieving your dream of reaching your ideal weight, you will want to immediately start searching to find the true deep-seated reason "why" you wish to lose weight. Develop your own personal process, one that's comfortable for you. I've found that it's very helpful to use a notebook, and then work on refining your "why" over a period of time, one step at a time. I just keep reading what I've written, and then keep "digging" deeper and deeper, to try to get to my true root feeling as to "why" I want to lose weight.

Find a quiet and comfortable place where you can do a little introspective thinking, and then write down all the reasons why it's important to you personally to lose weight, and there will probably be many reasons that come to your mind in the beginning. Start to prioritize your reasons "why", identifying which ones seem to be the most important to you, finally you'll start to see that some are just naturally rising to the top of your list; now you're starting to make some progress. Just be honest and true to yourself, this is all about you and no one else, so just keep digging. By doing this you will start to see that some are much more personal than others, and it's likely that those will be the more powerful ones, too.

When you finally find your true "why", it will stand "heads and shoulders" above the all of the others. Start working on this now, and you'll be off to a very good start. By paying close attention to your deepest inner feelings every day, you'll start to be able to refine your weight loss "why", and finally your true "why" will become clearly fixed in your mind. When this happens, you'll have the anchor that will virtually force you to keep yourself on your weight loss track, and it will become your source of personal motivation, one that will catapult your weight loss program forward.

This part is very important, so don't even think about skipping this step, or just settling on your first thought as to the reason "why" you want to achieve your weight loss. This step is absolutely critical to your success, so much so that I will unequivocally say that if you cheat yourself on this step, your chance for any positive long-term change in your weight will be next to impossible. I know that's a strong statement, but it's the truth, and being accountable to the truth is part of this program.

Let me try to add just a little more clarity to this in another way. Like it or not, everything we do, has a "why"

47

behind it. As I pointed out earlier, your current weight situation, your poor eating habits, your poor diet decisions and your excess eating, all have some sort of "why" buried behind each of them, too. Now, I'm not a psychologist, nor do I want to even spend five seconds trying to think about what those "whys" might be, it's not important because they are not going loosen their grasp on you all that easily. It's going to be up to you to push them out of your way by replacing them with your new stronger "why" that will support you're personal desire to be thin.

I want you to imagine that you're walking down a street, and that you're suddenly being faced by a bunch of mean spirited bullies, standing in your path; it makes it almost impossible to successfully move forward. But then the Sherriff shows up, and walks along beside you, and of course the bullies' scatter from sight. Well, just think of your weight loss "why" as your Sheriff, and how safe it makes you feel. Just be sure to keep the Sheriff at your side during your weight loss journey, and the weight-gain bullies will scatter like flies. As long as you keep your weight loss "why" at close hand, you're weight loss journey is insured to be safe, but let that Sheriff drift away, and you're bullies will surely return.

I believe that discovering your "why" will be the most powerful weight loss aid that you'll ever have. Your "why" will keep you on track when you feel like quitting, it will re-energize you when you've lost your enthusiasm, it will always be there to get you restarted in the right direction again. But, it's imperative that you find ways to keep your weight loss "why" clearly within your mind's vision, especially when you're actually eating, or around food in any fashion what so ever. Find your "why" and then work hard to firmly crystallize it within your mind; keep digging deeper for more clarity, keep refining it, and clarifying it. You're looking for that "why" that you instinctively know is important to you, and don't try to over think it, or to analyze what should be most important; your true "why" is the one that makes you feel

48

a special desire for losing your weight. The more clearly that you can see, and feel, that "why", the better you'll feel about being thin, and the more successful you'll be in achieving your desired weight loss. Your "why" is going to be your constant weight loss companion, your consistent reminder of the importance of forging past the obstacles, and past the discouragement, that you'll encounter. The best part of all of this is that it's completely up to you; you are worth it, and I know that you can do it!

Lastly, you're weight loss "why" is your secret, and it's something very personal to you, and to you alone. There is no right or wrong, as it's created from your own deep personal feelings and beliefs, it's yours and you have total ownership. Never feel any obligation to share your "why" with any one else, unless that's something you feel strongly that you want to do, and even then only do it cautiously, and only with those who you feel that you can absolutely trust to be unconditionally supportive. Perhaps even more importantly, never under any circumstances allow others to sit in judgment of your "why"; after all, it's your secret and it's none of their business, what so ever.

Dreams and Goals

Let's assume that you now have a clear picture as to "why" you truly want to lose weight, and to keep it off for the long term. That's great progress, but your "why" is simply the strength to keep on track, and to keep you pushing ahead. So, now it's time to start creating your plan; it's critical to have your "why" to keep you enthusiastically forging ahead, but you need to have a track to follow, and specific targets to achieve along your way to weight loss. This plan will be your own personal adventure, and it needs to be targeted to your specific personal objectives, those things that you want to accomplish along your path to weight loss. To do that, you'll need to look closely at your personal weight loss visions and dreams, because it's from those dreams that you'll develop your own specific personal goals, which in turn will become the track that leads you to your weight loss success. All of this will be designed and built by you, so that it provides you with exactly what you desire for your weight loss journey.

One of the things that I've learned from my many years in business is that setting good solid goals is a major key to achieving success in everything that we set out to accomplish. Our weight loss journey is no different, and it's our goals that will keep us on track, and headed directly toward achieving our ideal weight. I believe that the entire goal setting process can be fun. It starts first by identifying all of our wonderful dreams that relate to our long-term weight loss. Then, it's from those dreams that we will then start building a framework of goals that we'll follow, step by step, all the way to the final destination of our ideal weight.

Now, it's time to get out a pad and pencil again, because you're going to start writing down all of your dreams, and your visions for your future thinner self. This is your adventure, so be completely honest with yourself, and jot down everything that comes into your mind about your new thinness. Write down any dreams that you may have that relate to your weight loss, or your personal future thinness. It's these dreams that will become the foundation, for your new personal weight loss goals. Dream about how you want to look, how you will dress, how you will feel, the new fun things that you'll be doing, and the ways that your life will become better; and write down all of these dreams so that you don't allow these feelings to escape.

Take all of the time that you need, just sit back and close your eyes and imagine how you'll feel, and how you see yourself as you become thinner. Take a break, and then come back to it, and add the new dreams that have come into your mind. Write down your thoughts, your feelings, and whatever else it is that you desire to be doing in the future. Dream about your early stages of weight loss, as well as dreams that take you all the way to your new thinner self. Dream about how you'll look, and how you'll feel both during your weight loss journey, as well as when you've reached your desired target weight. Include your dreams for exercise, how exercise has become fun and how good you feel when doing new physical activities, and don't forget your dreams about how your body will become more toned each step of the way.

It's so very important that you capture all of your dreams in writing, as you don't want them to escape. Remember, these dreams are the foundation for your weight loss plan, and we are building a plan that is individually yours, one that will be built around your dreams, and your personal vision of the future. A plan that completely satisfies your weight loss "why" in every way, and makes you feel wonderful along the way. It's impossible for me to help you identify these personal dreams, so take the time right now to really indulge yourself in some full-fledged dreaming about your future self. No one has to see your list of dreams, no one will be passing judgment on them in any way whatsoever, these dreams are yours, and they are absolutely right simply because you chose them.

Okay, let's assume that you've begun your list of wonderful personal dreams, and that you've put them into a priority order, with the dreams that would naturally occur first, being the first ones on your list. It's these first dreams that will now become the foundation for your new weight loss goals, and which become the start of your weight loss plan. But, keep this list of dreams, as you will want to refer it many times in the coming months, plus you'll want to continue to make your dreams more specific, and to add new dreams to your list as your capabilities for weight loss dreaming naturally expands with your success.

So, let's get started with your goal setting process. Goals are very important for the success of your weight loss program, as they are the tracks that become your path; it's with these goals that you will be directing your actions, so that you can actually realize your dreams. Your personal weight loss plan is all about your dreams becoming your reality. Your goals become very motivational, and energizing, because they are yours personally, and they target those very things that you dream about.

Don't confuse these powerful personal goals with the kind of goals that may be handed out for your job at work. Those goals are really their goals, built around their company's dreams, not yours personally, and they are just trying to get you on track to embrace their goals plan. While those goals might be good for their business, they are rarely very motivational to employees. I bring this up simply so that you will understand that the kind of personal goals that we are talking about here, are totally focused on you, and have a significantly greater motivational power, than your goals at work.

The first step in developing your personal "weight loss goals program" is to identify one, or a few, of your short-term weight loss dreams. For example you might have had a short-term dream of being able to wear a certain piece of clothing, that's currently too tight, and uncomfortable. Okay, that makes it pretty simple, as you know from experience that if you knock off five pounds, those clothes will fit fine again. So now you develop some simple short-term actions steps that let you average losing one pound a week. I'm using this only as an example, as I feel it's an easily sustainable amount to lose, especially when first starting on your weight loss program.

I want to slow down here for a minute, and discuss the fact that everyone loses weight at a different rate, and in a different way. Even when two people follow identical diets, they almost always lose weight differently. There are many factors that affect weight loss, not the least is a person current weight, their height, body composition, gender, age, disease, medications, exercise level and more. Additionally, the correlation between weight loss, and body measurements is also different for everyone. For example one person may lose five pounds, and see a one-inch reduction in their waist size. Another person may require a greater weight loss to lose that same one-inch, and still another may require less. So, it's important to understand that when I give a weight loss example, it may, or may not be something that will work the same for you.

Using the above illustration, you'll lose five pounds in a five-week period, but let's make it six weeks, or longer, just to make it easy for starters. You see, these goals are your goals, so you can set them any way that you want, and you can move ahead at a faster pace, or slower, whatever is best for you. You can change your plan at any time you wish, if that's what you want to do. Just be sure that you move forward with your weight loss at a healthy, and sensible pace, and to be sure that you know what rate of weight loss will be healthy for you, be sure to check with your medical professional.

This is your very own personally designed program, and that's why it's going to work for you; but you still have more to do. In order for your goals to provide you with truly powerful motivation, they must be in writing, and be written as a specific positive statement, made in the first person. This is very important, as this is your way of making your goals inescapable. Remember that we said earlier that your weight loss success was dependant upon your being accountable, so here is an example of how you'll be accountable to yourself. But there's more, and that's the fact that there's nothing to be accountable for if your goals do not have realistic deadlines for their attainment.

Now with your pen in hand, and following your list of weight loss dreams, you will start to create the first of your specifically written personal weight loss goals. You'll want these goals to be achievable steps toward the realization of your dreams; they will all need to be stated positively, in the first person, and each with a deadline for their attainment. If one of your dreams is a really big dream, then you'll want to develop a series of smaller goals that will in turn lead you to the achievement of your larger goal, and dream. In other words, for each and every dream, you'll be developing a specific plan of action that will see each dream through to reality, and be achieved in the time frame that you choose. Goals must always be in writing, and be made as a positive statement in the first person. As examples: "I will weigh 150 pounds on (date)"; or, "I will fit comfortably into my white gown by (date)".

I said earlier in this book, you're going to need to "keep you eye on the ball", so as you move forward, your real focus will be on the very next specific goal on your list; this is all about taking one small step at a time, not trying to rush to the final end.

You'll use this goal setting process throughout your entire weight loss program. At first, you'll set small achievable goals; each goal should build one upon another. Soon you'll find that you've achieved a lot, and you'll have done it one small step at a time. Please don't be afraid of making a mistake, this is you're plan and you can do it the way you want, but if you find yourself faced with a goal that seems too big, just keep in mind that you can break it down in to smaller goals at any time, and as you begin to achieve those smaller goals, you'll soon be back on track. As you move ahead along your path to weight loss success, you'll find yourself building new, and larger, goals because you can now see that they too, are achievable.

In the beginning, not everyone finds goal setting to be an easy process, especially if goal setting is new, and you have yet to build strong faith in the power of goals to help you reach your personal objectives. In the past, perhaps you've felt somewhat powerless over your weight situation, if you have, you'll find that your new goals will empower you, and provide you with new confidence that your weight loss objectives are truly achievable.

Going back to our first example, where you've set a goal to lose five pounds, that's a great goal and a great place to start. Start working on your dreams and goals now, and don't worry if they're not perfect right from the start. Over time you'll modify your goals many times, to fit your most current dreams, which will have continued to expand. As that happens, you will have become successful in achieving your smaller support goals, and you'll naturally start setting new bigger goals for yourself. You're begin to build an entire framework of short-term goals, goals that you'll achieve one at a time, and all of which will lead the way to your achieving your ultimate long-term weight loss goals.

It's natural that you'll find some goals that you'll want to adjust and change. This is normal, and will continue throughout the entire process as your mind becomes more able to conceive of even bigger dreams. As your goals become more specific, and your deadlines more realistic, your goals will soon become reality. This reality will energize you even more as you move toward your ultimate weight loss goal, after all these were your dreams and goals, so their realization will be a truly rewarding reality.

Don't worry that you still have little idea about what your personal diet plan, or exercise plan, will look like; we'll get to that soon. Before you get to that point, you'll want to have a good understanding of your specific goals. After all, how can you realistically establish a new eating regiment, until you have a crystal clear vision as to where your dietary plan is supposed to take you, and how fast? And, that's why you'll be designing your own actual diet, and your own exercise plan, and doing it in concert with your specific dreams and goals; and you'll be adjusting them along the way, as you move forward on your weight loss journey. Soon, you'll see how this all fits together, and how you will have built yourself an empowering personal plan for weight loss success.

Putting Your Plan Into "Warp Drive"

The real strength and stability behind your weight loss success will always be your "why", as it's your own very powerfully motivating secret. On this weight loss journey, it's your "why" that provides your power and stability, and it's what will keep you moving steadily forward toward your next goal, and to your weight loss destination. We've all seen railroad tracks, and how they seem to lead off to somewhere, but we've also seen the locomotives, and box cars, just sitting on the tracks and going nowhere. Your goals may be your tracks, but you need power in order to pick up speed, and keep moving forwards down your tracks. Trains start very slowly, and then build up speed until they're finally roaring down the tracks toward their destination, and that's how it is with goal setting, too.

Goals absolutely do work, and they will work for everyone, but when you're new to goal setting, and just starting out toward your destination, you'll only be able to move forward at the rate that your beliefs allow you, as it's your belief that powers your goals. Goal setting is a long-term process, and by taking one small step at a time your confidence will build, and your steps will become easier. When you finally have complete belief in your goals, and they've become clearly and firmly set within your mind, your weight loss "train" will then be going full speed down your goal track, directly toward the achievement of your ideal weight.

With that said, it's critical to understand that as you move through life, your dreams and desires will naturally evolve, and because of this your "why", and your goals, are both likely to change some, too. Your long-term weight loss plan is a lifetime commitment, and it will always be up to you to continually be in touch with your most current desires, and feelings. And, from those feelings you'll want to regularly be updating your deepest weight loss "why", along with your supporting goals. The simple fact is that your long-term weight loss is not a destination; it's not simply a place where you arrive. Your long-term weight loss is a continuing journey that you must travel throughout your life.

It's one thing to find your "why", and to set your goals, but it's yet another for you to completely accept them deep within your belief system, and believe that they can actually be achieved by you. Let me emphasize again that your "why", and your goals, are totally yours; they've been created by you and for you, and when you have absolute belief in them, they will bring you the strength and desire that you need to propel you to your weight loss success. Your goals and your "why" are your two best friends, and they will keep you centered on your path to weight loss; they tell you where you're going, and "why" you're going there. Still, with everything else that goes on in our lives, sometimes our newly seated beliefs can slowly drift from our focus, and it's imperative that we make sure that does not happen. There are three valuable things that we can do, which can help us keep properly focused, add power to our goals and build commitment to our "why". Those powerful things are (1) the embracing of our "why", (2) our affirmations, and (3) our visualizations.

Embracing your "why", Affirmations and Visualizations

You've identified your "why", and you have some very good personal reasons for choosing that "why". Because your "why" is the secret that gives you powerful weight loss motivation, let's find ways to make it even more motivating. A great way to do that is by immediately involving yourself in as many aspects of your why, as possible. Take time every day, maybe even a few times every day, to research and find out everything you can that relates to your "why". The more can become emotionally involved with all aspects of your "why", the more powerful it will be in supporting your weight loss. For example, let's say that you have a "why" to be trim and fit enough to go on regular twenty mile mountain hikes. So, if that's your "why", you'll want to start buying hiking magazines, learning about new and different mountain trails, and checking out all of the interesting hiking equipment that's available on the market. And, don't forget to investigate all of the nice hiking clothes that you'll be able to wear, with your new trim body. Start taking short walks, and then short hikes, allowing them to become longer as you progress with your weight loss program. Completely immerse yourself in every aspect of your "why", as by doing this you'll create lasting enthusiasm, and your commitment will become stronger and stronger. Perhaps this example is not at all like your own personal "why", but hopefully you get the idea, and can see how very important this aspect of your weight loss program can be for you.

Next, affirmations are a powerful way to support your "why", and your goals. And, they are strategic reminders as to "why" you feel that your weight loss success is so important to you. Many people have found it to be very helpful to use written affirmations to support their beliefs, and provide power for their goals. Some carry these positive statements in their pocket so they are at hand all the time, some put them around the house or on the refrigerator door, others will have written affirmations affixed to their bathroom mirror, computer, automobile dashboard, and other convenient places where these affirmations become constant reminders that support their goals, and their "why". It's even more important to try to keep these affirmations close to you, when you're around food. Possibly, you could even carry a small token in your pocket that remained you of your "why", and then place it next to your plate when eating. Anything like that, which works for you, will be a very helpful and supportive reminder for you when eating, and when you're around food.

Affirmations for your goals might sound something like these: "I only eat when I'm hungry", or "I eat slowly", or "When I get hungry between meals, I snack only on fruits and vegetables", or any other supportive positive statement that supports the weight loss goals that you've set for yourself.

Affirmations for your "why" might sound something like these: "I am slim and trim; a great example of good health for my children to follow", or "I feel wonderful wearing new slim styled clothing", (or name whatever else it may be that embodies your "why"). Your affirmations may be as long or as short as you'd like them to be, because they are simply positive supportive statements that are meaningful to you, and that specifically affirm "why" your feeling happy about heading toward your new thinness.

As it is with your goals, it's imperative that your affirmations be stated only as a positive statement, never negatively, and be stated in the first person. Affirmations will slowly infiltrate your subconscious mind, and will provide you with strong support. But, your subconscious mind is not capable of judging right from wrong, or good from bad; it takes in whatever you feed into it, so it's important that you always clearly state your affirmations in a positive fashion, so that they will provide positive reinforcement for your weight loss plan.

There's a second kind of affirmation, and it's one that's perhaps your most powerful force for change; it's the "self-talk" affirmation. "Self-talk" is the technique of feeding your mind with your own verbal positive affirmations statements. Find a place where you can speak out loud to yourself, and then state your positive affirmations so that you can actually hear your own voice saying the words; and try to speak in front of a mirror so that you can see yourself saying them too. By doing this regularly, you'll find that your confidence, and your belief in yourself, will begin to strengthen and soar. For self-talk to truly be effective, it's very important to speak your affirmations out loud so that you can actually hear yourself saying the words, you may feel self-conscious in the beginning, but that will soon pass and you'll start to feel comfortable, and it will even become enjoyable. The wonderful thing about "self-talk", and why it's so powerful, is that there is no other person in the world that we trust more than ourselves, so when we regularly tell ourselves that we can do something, it is easy to see why our subconscious minds accept that as absolute fact. So, start telling yourself that you love the feeling of being thin; you won't believe the difference that this small act will make in your life. Again, I can't overstate how important it is that your "self-talk" be stated only as a positive statement that affirms your "why", and your goals for success.

Visualization is another extraordinarily powerful way to keep yourself anchored, and your goals on track. Visualization is simply a visual affirmation. For example, a picture showing the way that you might like to look at your target weight could make a powerful visualization of the weight loss objective that you seek to achieve. Cut some pictures from a magazine that show people the way you'll look when you've lost your weight, and keep the pictures where you can see them, to help you keep focused. As stated before, perhaps a token that you keep with you when you eat, would serve as a good visualization aid. Personally, I have a specially created picture of me that has my head superimposed on another man's very trim body. It may not be realistic, and it's sort of "cutesy", nevertheless I keep it by the mirror in my bathroom, and I see myself that way every day. There are many possibilities for strong visualization assistance for supporting both your "why", and your goals, just be creative and be sure that they portray a positive visual picture. Actually seeing, or visualizing, the end result of your goal track, will be an extraordinarily powerful aid in reaching your goal.

Before we continue, I want to say that I recognize that we've moved quickly through a lot of material, and that much of it may have been new to you. I'd like to emphasize that this is all very important, and it's going to be well worth your time to re-read this section as many times as you need. Don't feel overwhelmed by all of this;

this is your plan, and your time schedule, so move at the pace that's most comfortable for you. Please remember that there's nothing that you can do, that you can't easily adjust or correct later, if need be. Just move ahead, one small step at a time; the real key is for you to just keep going.

Building New Habits

Earlier, I identified a number of obvious poor eating habits, and asked that you also make a list of your own poor eating habits. This list is important because you need to identify those things that are working against your weight loss goals. Getting rid of bad habits is extraordinarily difficult, and seemingly almost impossible at times. The good news is that there's a way to change your bad habits. Although the process may seem simple, it's not always easy, nor is a permanent result likely to be achieved quickly. Nevertheless, your poor eating habits must change, if you're going to meet your new weight loss goals.

The process of eliminating poor eating habits is one of replacing your old poor habits, with new good habits. Repetitious behavior creates habits; our recurring actions eventually become embedded within our mind as a habit. Rather than to expect that we can make old habits just go away, it's much more efficient to teach ourselves new good habits, and to then allow those new habits to replace the old ones. Using a few of our previous examples, let's look at how this might work.

Eating Too Fast: Start making it a practice to set your fork, or spoon, down between each bite. Or, you might decide to silently count to a number like 10 or 15, between each bite.

Taking Second Helpings: Give yourself a "proper" first helping, and then remove the serving bowl to another location so that it's out of your easy reach, and out of temptation. If the habit of taking second helpings is hard for you stop, then you might think about using a smaller serving plate, and taking two smaller half-size portions. Remember that you're your own "food police", so you need to be honest and accountable in the judging of your portion sizes.

Eating Everything On Your Plate: If this is something that you feel that you've been doing automatically, as a habit, then start to eat only part of the food on your plate every time you eat. Start to build the habit of always leaving something on your plate, and you'll soon find it easy to stop eating when you're no longer hungry. Yes, it is okay to leave food on your plate!

Drinking Regular (Sugar) Soda Pop: Substitute a zero calorie soft drink, but if that's nutritionally unacceptable to you, there are many other alternatives such as water with lemon, iced tea or a lower calorie fruit juice, all of which are readily available.

Continual Snacking: No matter if you call it "emotional eating", "eating out of habit", "feel good eating", or just plain "snacking", the behavior can be very complicated, and a serious weight loss issue. One simple solution is to eliminate treats from your easy access, which can help, but personally I don't think that really cuts to the heart of the issue with most people. I say that because I've fought this issue most of my life, and I've found that boredom can be one of the biggest causes for this constant "snacking". When you're bored or relatively inactive, like when watching television, browsing the Internet or other such things, you are at much greater risk for impulse eating. Times like these, when you're not as physically active as you could be, are an open invitation for habitual "snacking" and "feel good eating". The key is to replace that inactivity with new and enjoyable physical activities. Do anything that keeps you active, go for a walk, go to the gym, do chores around the house, find a new hobby, take a second job, or participate in some group or sports activity; just be doing something that you enjoy that's active, and non-sedentary. You will not only reduce your opportunity for easy snacking, you'll also get extra physical activity, and reap big weight loss dividends. Put these kinds of activities on your goals list.

As you can easily see from these few examples, it's fairly easy to figure out a workable substitute for virtually every poor eating habit. Remember, the task is not simply one of determining what the substitute habit might be, but it's one of you being accountable for actually making the substitutions on a steady recurring basis. You will always have your personal "why", and your goals to help support you with consistently purging your old poor eating habits, and replacing them with better new habits.

Attitude Is Everything

It is unfortunate that some of us actually come to a new dietary plan, with less than a positive attitude. Sometimes we allow our attitudes to be shaped by outside influences, and quite often that includes advertising, news media, movies, television and more. Without question fast food advertisers seek to make it glamorous, and fun, to eat their high calorie food concoctions, most often loaded with salt, sugar and fat. Advertisements from "sit-down" restaurants promote their indulgent menus, and large portions. Advertisements like this can soon create the image in our minds that these kinds of foods are the norm, and therefore acceptable for us to eat. Although it may be difficult at times, maintaining a positive healthy attitude about your weight loss, and staying within the constraints of your self-constructed dietary plan, is important for your success.

Positive attitudes can be developed and practiced, and to do so it's important build a natural pattern of positive behavior. Taking positive actions, and having positive thoughts, will create positive attitudes. I suggest replacing negative words and phrases, with positive ones. Replace "I can't" with the phrase "I can"; "If" with the word "When"; "I don't have the time" with the phrase "I will make the time"; "Maybe" with the phrase

"Positively"; and, "I doubt" with the phrase "I'm confidant". In general try to avoid all negative words, especially words like, no, not, can't, don't and won't.

Making small positive changes like these in your everyday behavior will pay you big dividends, not only toward the achievement of your weight loss goal, but also in every other area of your life. When you have a positive attitude it becomes contagious, and will be inspirational to those around you, and they will start to become more positive, too. Positive attitudes are the cornerstone of all successes, and your weight loss success is no different. The more people that you have around you that are also positive, the more positive you'll become, too; positive attitudes beget positive attitudes. On a similar note, when you show enthusiasm for everything that you are doing, you will inspire others around you to also become enthusiastic. You will find that having both enthusiasm, and positivity, will improve your weight loss success drastically.

Tracking Your Results

Earlier we had a section called, "Cop-Outs" that we hear and use, and it covered a little bit about excuses that have become so prevalent in the world of eating. An excuse is nothing more than an outward expression of the lack of accountability. The topic of accountability has been covered at some length in the other sections of this book, but lack of accountability of one's self, is a primary cause for the collapse and failure of weight loss plans. Specifically, failing to be accountable for over eating, eating the wrong foods, and the lack of exercise are all obvious accountability issues.

Make no mistake about it, every long-term successful weight loss program, has a component of hard work, dedication and personal accountability. And, the only effective way to combat excuses, and the accompanying lack of accountability, is by tracking the results of both your weight loss success, as well as your specific weight loss activities; by doing this you now have an inescapable record of your ongoing actual results. Your tracking must be done regularly, and in writing (or computer), so that all of your actual progress is clearly visible. Normally, if your plan starts to slide off track, it is because your tracking, and your accountability have become lax. If, or when, that happens, immediately get back to tracking everything, and that means writing everything down, just the way you did when you started. The only person that you're accountable to, for the results achieved by your weight loss plan is you.

Then There's Sleep

There appears to be mounting evidence showing that getting rest, namely a good night's sleep, is beneficial for healthy weight loss. I would suggest that if you have interest in learning more about the importance of sleep that you do some research on your own. It is my personal belief that any time that you make a change in your life, especially a change in the way you think about things, or a change in your habits, it creates a certain amount of stress and anxiety. One of the best ways to relieve that stress is through rest, and especially by getting good sound sleep. Because of this, I highly recommend that as part of your new weight loss program that you also establish goals for getting enough rest each day.

Section VII
Let's Get You Started

Two and half years ago, I again found myself at 265, and I knew that something had to be done. Having been through a lifetime of dieting, I had a pretty good feel for what worked for me, and what didn't. At the time my wife was attending "Weight Watchers®", but I knew that the "group meeting" setting wasn't for me. I'm a pretty independent sort of person, so I really wanted to customize something for myself, and have it be focused on what I wanted to eat. Earlier, my wife had told me about a website called www.Sparkpeople.com, so I went to that site and as it turns out, the site is extremely comprehensive, focused entirely upon weight loss, exercise and good health. For me, the best part was the fact that it was free, I like that. I had already established a pretty clear mindset that the major key to losing weight was managing my caloric intake, on a meal-by-meal and a day-to-day basis. I also found that Sparkpeople.com could help me to analyze my dietary calorie requirements, which is something that had always been missing before. I'd read a lot about calorie consumption, and the per-day requirements for different types of people, but in that we're all so different, those preset calorie calculations just never seemed quite right to me; I was happy to find something that could help me customize that part of the equation. The site could also track my day-to-day food intake activity, and that's something that I still use the site for today.

There are many other websites that will do much the same thing as SparkPeople.com. One site that I also like is MyFitnessPal.com, which is free and has a free mobile application too, for those who like using mobile devices. Then there's the "Weight Watchers®" site, which also has a mobile application, but I don't believe that either of those "Weight Watchers®" sites are free. For those interested, there's also a free iPhone application that I sometimes use for scanning bar codes in the grocery stores. That site is "Healthy Diet & Grocery Food

Scanner", by ShopWell™, and it can easily be found in iTunes. I encourage you to find a good website, one that you're comfortable with, and will contain the same useful weight, measurement, and exercise tracking tools. Most of these websites will also have a lot of useful recipe recommendations, and even a blog where you can communicate with others about your weight loss activities.

I knew that it was mandatory for me to be accountable, and that I must track both what I ate each day as well as my weight loss progress. The website has been useful for me in tracking my calories, body measurements and my weight loss; it provided me with all of the tools necessary for me to stay on the specific track that I set for myself. For me, this seemed like the perfect tool to aid my weigh loss journey.

I've also found that having an accurate scale for weighing myself is helpful, and because everyone's weight tends to fluctuate on a day-to-day basis, I personally weigh myself only once a week, and at the same time of day; and, I'd recommend that you do the same. If you choose to track your body measurements, that's sort of fun because as you start to lose the weight, you also start to see your actual sizes drop, too. In tracking your measurements (measure what's most important to you), you'll find that sometimes even though you may not have achieved a weekly weight loss (it does happen), you may still have had an improvement in a measurement, which is still great encouragement. Additionally, I purchased a small, inexpensive, electronic food scale; that way I could start to weigh my food on a meal-by-meal basis, and by doing that I could accurately determine the proper food portions for my plan. I started carrying a small notepad with me too. I carried it wherever I went, even around the house so I could write down everything that I ate all day, every day; that insured that I wouldn't lose track of the things I snacked on.

Many of the foods that I chose to include in my personal weight loss plan were inspired by the information that I'd learned from the previously mentioned book, "Dine Out and Lose Weight". It was from that book that I learned a lot about complex carbohydrates, and which vegetables were the most weight loss friendly. This was helpful for me, as I enjoy eating many vegetables, and it was helpful in devising my own dietary regiment, which allowed me to eat pretty much whatever I wanted. Of course, I had to adjust some the quantities from what I'd been used to eating, so that they matched my daily calorie allotment. For me, this is a lot better than following someone else's plan that tries to tell me what I should eat, as those plans rarely include the things that I like to eat.

I quickly learned that certain vegetables could fill me up without using up too much of my calorie allotment. I also learned that by aggressively trimming the fat from many of the meats, I was able cut their calorie count down to much more acceptable numbers. It's not that these were new concepts to me, it's just that now that I was actually being accountable, and weighing pretty much everything I was eating, and that's when all of this became much more obvious to me.

Initially, I did a lot of research on the different foods I liked, and I got really good at learning the calorie contents by reading the ingredient labels in the stores. I also used the Internet to search for caloric information, too. You can go to the search engine of your choice, and enter the word calories, along with the name of whatever kind of food that you're curious about, and you'll find that it's a great resource. When reading food packaging, it's important to be sure to calculate the serving number, along with the number of calories, to accurately know what various food packages contain. I look at it like a game, where the food supplier doesn't want to show too many calories, so they keep the calorie number low, by increasing their number of projected servings shown on the packaging. For example I saw some frozen pizzas in the grocery store the other day, one said 330 calories and

3 servings (990 calories), the other (same size and brand) with a different topping showed 340 calories, but 4 servings (1,360 calories). Like I say, it's a game, but I don't make these rules, I just try to play their game to my benefit. It can be confusing, and if you're not too good with math, you might want to carry a small calculator with you to the store. Don't be afraid to play their "calorie game", start making your shopping fun by checking calories in everything, you'll start to enjoy it, and soon you will have learned a lot.

As I said earlier, the website that I use allows me to enter my weight loss goal, and how long I want to take to achieve that goal. It then factors in my age, sex, weight, and activity level. This gives me an estimate for the approximate number of calories necessary for me to eat each day, in order to achieve that goal. Although I found this to be very helpful, I also found that initially I'd been a little conservative on my original goal projections, and it was therefore relatively easy for me to achieve a lower caloric intake than I'd set up in the plan. I point this out only to illustrate that continual "tweaking" of the plan will be needed before you feel that you have a plan that's totally comfortable for you. Of course, there are always some days when I eat more than my daily calorie allowance, but for the most part I pretty much stay close, or just under the projections.

The result of this day-by-day monitoring, and tracking, was the achievement of about 40 pounds of weight loss, dropping my weight to near 225 pounds. I feel that the reason for my success in staying with this diet plan for so long was that I was able to easily track my daily calories, and that allowed me to see the ongoing impact of my weight loss plan. I had no regulation as to the kinds of food that I ate, and from time to time I pretty much ate everything that I liked; my only regulation was on my calories. This meant that many of the things that I ate had to be eaten with substantial moderation, but sometimes I chose to adjust the size of other meals in the day, to accommodate a larger meal that I wanted to eat, and that kind of moderation worked well for me, too. Needless to say, learning moderation is key for all weight loss. I felt that my self-devised plan was a success, because the plan was designed by me, to specifically fit my own personal "wants", and because the plan was carefully tracked and closely self-regulated. It was great, but I still had not gotten everything clearly figured out the way I knew that I must.

Over time, I again slipped in my eating habits, and I found myself back to more than 240 pounds, which meant that I'd given up about half of my previous weight loss. On one hand, I didn't find this situation particularly depressing, because I felt like my self-designed weight loss plan was still in place, it had worked for me before, and it could easily be restarted. On the other hand, I decided to do some more work on how to rid myself of the dreaded yo-yo effect that seems to plague us all. That was when I decided to look to my past business experience, I wanted to find something that was proven to work, and that's when I discovered the missing piece; understanding my "why".

Good business always has a clearly defined reason "why" that sits at the root of each and every goal. And, that's when it hit me that a focused weight loss "why" was what was missing. It's not that I had no idea why I wanted to lose weight, of course I did. But, it was really a very shallow "why" that I'd never really taken any time to truly focus on. The fact was, I didn't have a "why" that was anywhere close to being a super-solid, long-lasting reason for "why" I specifically wanted to permanently lose weight. Honestly, I think that we all just feel that we naturally know why we want to lose weight, and we just take that for granted. Some may feel that the difference seems small, but my business experience has taught me that you'd better always have a strong reason "why" behind what you're doing, or your success just won't "stick".

Let me give you a business example. Think about this, let's just say that doing a task that you've done many times before, and suddenly the big boss comes up to you and asks you, "Why are you doing it that way?" You know that if you say to the boss, "This is how I've always done it", it's not very likely that you'll get a favorable response. Yet on the other hand, if your response to the boss shows that you have a clearly defined reason "why" you're doing it that way, and that reason "why" makes it clear to the boss that you have a clear vision of the boss's business goals, then your answer will make you look very good. And, so it is with weight loss, if you just follow a diet plan like a robot, without having a clearly defined super-solid long-lasting reason "why", then the diet plan is not likely to have much ability to sustain your weight loss for the long-term.

Since that time, I've worked very hard to refining my own personal "why", and I've made surprising new progress. Although I'd originally thought that I knew "why" I wanted to lose weight, I found that I'd not dug deeply enough to fully uncover my deepest and strongest "why". In fact what I eventually found is that the "whys" that I first thought to be the most straight-forward and logical, were not at all the ones that were deeply motivating to me. The reality is that our own deep feelings, and emotions, can be substantially different from what we may logically think. And, it's only the true "why", the one that's derived from our deep-seated emotional feelings and experiences that will actually have the motivational power we seek in support of our weight loss. Again, I want to stress that this weight loss journey is personally yours, your "why" is your own, and it's right simply because you've found it to be the thing that's so deeply important to you personally. There is no need to share this with anyone, ever. In fact I'd recommend that you think about not sharing your "why" with anyone; it's my belief is that the better you protect you personal "why" from the possible critique of others, the better off you'll be in your weight loss journey. You're losing weight for you, and not for anyone else.

Now that my "why" is much more specifically defined, I feel more enthusiastic than ever about my weight loss plan, and I'm again making the slow methodical progress set out by my personal plan. I'm no different than you, and I continue to work on all of my dreams and goals, which keeps me energized and optimistic about my weight loss journey. I now have my own clear personal path to long-term weight loss success; my "why" has cleared the path for me, and my goals have given me the track to follow.

Enough about my story, let's get you started on your own path to weight loss success. You've stuck with me this far, which makes me very excited about your future success, too.

Researching Food For Your Own Custom Diet

There's no way that I'm I going to try to tell you what to eat, how much to eat or when to eat, all of that is going to be up to you. We will discuss how you might best go about making your diet choices, but those choices must be your own, or you'll soon drop away from this plan, just like others in the past. This is a long-term approach for taking control of your own eating habits, your weight and your future. It goes without saying that such a program will subject you to many eating changes, including continual changes in your diet. This will happen because certain foods will become boring for you, and new foods will become attractive. And, finally there will be more change when you slowly convert from your weight loss diet plan, to your maintenance diet plan.

In managing your diet plan, you're going to need some help along the way. Thankfully, we have the Internet as a resource, so that will be where you get a major portion of the information that you'll need. Almost every day I'm looking up how many calories that there are in some new food, looking for new low calorie recipes, and other miscellaneous things that might help me keep my caloric intake low, while still allowing my food to taste good. I also spend a fair amount of time checking out restaurant menu items that might work for me, I do this particularly for the fast food restaurants, and it's amazing what I learn. These restaurants have come a long way in acknowledging the potential business of "calorie counters" like us. For example "McDonald's®" has a page on their site that shows all of their menu items that are under 400 calories, I recently counted forty-four items on that page, with about 17 of them being entrée items, with the others being things like diet coke, and etc. Burger King®, offers a nice spreadsheet type layout that shows you everything, as does "Jack in the Box®", "KFC®" and others, but unfortunately, some of them have the print so small it can't easily be read; I'm a little cynical, and personally suspect that this is done on purpose so that it's hard to see that most of their food items are loaded with calories.

The Federal Government now has regulations in place that require all restaurants, with twenty or more locations, to post their nutritional information. The competitive nature of the restaurant business seems to also be encouraging many of the smaller competing restaurants to also post their information, even though it's not required. This kind of nutritional information is the kind of thing you'll want to start paying very close attention to, as you start working to fit only a certain number of calories into your daily diet. If you're like me, you'll want to be sure that you use your calories by eating only the foods you like best. I've also learned that by simply asking most restaurants for their calorie information, that many will quickly produce it for you; watching your calories when eating out is getting easier every day. As a last thought on this subject, some restaurants make it hard to locate their calorie information on their website, so I've found that searching the Internet using the restaurant name along with the word nutritional, or nutrition, works pretty well for finding most of the illusive information.

Now, let's discuss some of the prepared plans that exist, such as "Jenny Craig®", NutriSystem®, SlenderZone® and many more; some national and some local. Honestly I've never tried any of these systems for three reasons. First, I want to choose what I eat, and how it's prepared. Second, it would cost me more than buying, and cooking, my own food. And third, their plans are basically weight loss plans, and although they may also have "maintenance meals", in the long run eating those same meals regularly would likely get very boring, as well as expensive. With that said, I respect that many people have very busy schedules that make cooking meals difficult, and some have families that will want full calorie meals, which might not work for those individuals who are on a weight loss plan. It's hard to cook separate sets of meals for different groups of people. Perhaps prepared plans like these have some merit for those situations, either as a full menu, or as a supplement menu. The bottom line is that if any of these plans will work for you, fit within the weight loss guidelines that you've set for yourself, and have foods you like, then there's probably nothing wrong with utilizing them when it benefits you.

In addition to the prepared meal plans, there's also the "Weight Watchers®" system, and numerous other similar systems promoting a myriad of different "benefits". I've attended a "Weight Watchers®" meeting, I've studied much of their material and I've known numerous people who have found their plan successful. One nice thing about "Weight Watchers®" is that their website, http://www.weightwatchers.com, has lots of recipes, and other stuff for free even if you don't join their plan. They also have a web based weight loss program, where you don't have to attend one of their meetings if your schedule, or your personality, is not meeting friendly, but this plan does have a fee. I will say that "Weight Watchers®" seems to have a very sound, consistent and education-based program that I know has been successful for many people.

I have not seen, or tried all of the "fee based" weight loss programs that exist, and there are a lot of them. But, I have no reason to think that there's a need to avoid them, if it's what you feel you want to do. With that said, however, anytime you start utilizing a diet that doesn't contain the specific foods that you like, you have a great risk of eventually falling away from that plan. And, regardless of whatever diet plan you use, keeping your weight loss "why" close at hand will always be important to your success.

I have one last thing to say about my food and calorie research. I originally had the idea to try to list every website that could be useful in researching food calories, menu items and etc. But, I soon realized that not only were there too many sites to list, they also changed constantly so that any list would soon become worthless. Instead, I want to suggest a few phrases that you can put into the search engine of your choice, and which are likely to help you find sites with useful information. Of course some will be tying to sell something, but you'll be surprised at how many sites exist that have valuable free information. Here are some possible search phrases, which you may find useful, and of course you can find many more of your own, too.

Finding Food Ideas On The Internet

Calorie free cooking
Calories in (name any food you like)
Cooking sugar free
Diet recipes
Food and calorie information websites
Food calorie research
Low calorie diets
Low calorie Italian recipes
       (substitute any other type of food you like)
Low calorie meals
Low calorie recipes
Low carbohydrate meals
Low fat meals

I think that you get the idea; you'll be surprised at the wealth of information available to you when you make use of the Internet by just asking good questions. Soon you will start to build your own information base of good sites, and you'll find some really good foods that you like to eat, all of which will put you securely onto your path to weight loss success.

Getting Your Plan Started; You're New Beginning

Let's get you started on setting up your system, and creating an outline, for your weight loss program. If you like, you can do this by using a notebook, a computer or an online system of your choice. You'll want to decide which things are most important for you to track, and decide the best way for you to track things like your food and calorie consumption by meal, your weekly weight change, your body measurements, how much water you drink each day, perhaps various nutritional factors in your diet, and more. As you get down the road on this plan, you may want to make some adjustments on what you track, and how often, so keep that kind of flexibility in mind when you set up your system. Then there's your exercise component, so you'll also want to decide how you're going to track your physical activates, things like what activities you are doing, when and for how long.

You already have some idea as to what your weight loss goal will be, so it's best to start by using that, although you may decide to adjust that at a later time. Now you'll need to do some research to determine the maximum number of calories you want to consume each day. This will vary based on your sex, age, current weight, your target weight and the time period in which you'd like to achieve your weight loss goal. And, as you get started on the plan, it's very likely that you'll want to adjust some of these factors, as it's very important that you "tweak" your plan so that it's absolutely customized to fit your situation, and your personal desires. If you do less than that, you'll end up with a plan that you're not happy with, and that you'll likely not be willing to stick with. Needless to say, that's a rather overwhelming task, but don't let that deter you. All of this is a lot simpler than it sounds, but it will require your attention in the beginning in order to get it all set up correctly. Just keep in mind the importance of the process, it's all about creating a new, better, healthier and happier you. The effort that you put in setting up this plan, will pay you big dividends down the road when you have a plan that works easily, and smoothly, and totally fits your life style.

It's my recommendation that you go to the Internet, and search for "Free web based diet management plans"; why pay for one when you can get one for free? You will find pages of results, many of them quite good sites. Or, as I said earlier, my favorite site, and the one that I've been using for quite a while, is the free website www.SparkPeople.com; just so you know, I have absolutely no affiliation with this site, I just like it and that's why I recommend it. As far as I'm concerned this site offers everything that you'll need, like a way to make all of the calculations that I outlined above, a system where you can modify those factors whenever you want. It has lots of useful weight loss ideas and information, recipes, tracking and even blogs by the members. I really like the fact that the site is easy to use, and that you can easily set up your own customized plan, which can be totally adjusted at any time. One feature that I make a lot of use of is their "Favorites" tab, where I can enter, and save, my favorite foods, making it easy to log them into my personal tracking with one click, whenever I eat them. It makes the system very personalized, but it's also handy that there are a lot of other general food items that have already been pre-listed into the system; it's all pretty simple, once you're past a short learning curve. There are a lot of other features, including an automatic graphing component that visually shows your progress in weight, body measurements, and for exercise. I find it a very easy site to use, and believe me, I'm not a "techie"; if it's complicated, I look elsewhere.

Let's assume that you've decided to use a website to calculate, and track, your weight loss plan, and that you've chosen the site that you'll be using. First you'll want to go to the website and look around at the various pages and tabs, look for a section that shows you how to get started, and then experiment a little on the site so that you're familiar with its capabilities and how it works. Once you've done that, and feel confidant that this site will work for you, then start by entering in all of your current information, so that you have the site all set up the way that you want it to be.

The next part is sort of fun, as you'll want to start to experiment with some of the different combinations of weight loss amounts, and the time periods for that weight loss, in order to determine the best combination for you. I realize that at this point, you may not have any idea just how many calories a day will comfortably work for you, and knowing that is important. The program will be able to project different scenarios, based on different weight loss versus time periods that you input, so you'll just want to fool around with that for a while, and do your best to find the right starting place for you. For example, you may wish to initially set the your plan up so it's a short term plan to knock off your first five or ten pounds, and then reset your plan for your next intermediate goal. Personally, I prefer to set it up for my long-term goal, even if the weight loss period ends up being a year, or more. For me, the thing that's important is finding the right balance between being able to eat enough calories to feel comfortable, while still being able to lose weight; the time period (for me) is less important, as I'm in it for the long-term.

Once you get started, you'll begin to get a "feel" for what eating regiment you're comfortable with, and what you're not. Personally, I have learned that for my age, height, current weight, and activity level I can be comfortable with a calorie level of from 1150, to 1350 calories per day. Of course your plan will be different than mine, as it will be uniquely yours. In setting up your weight loss goals, I would be sure to adjust your time period, and your target weight, so that your projected calories for a given day are both comfortable and effective for your weight loss. It's important that you maintain your calories at a comfortable and manageable level, as that will give you your best chance for success. It is better to have a plan that you're able to stick with, even if it takes a longer period to lose your weight, than it is to have a plan that you dislike, and then consequently drop away from altogether.

Weight Loss Ideas To Explore

Now that you're organized, with the framework for managing your customized weight loss program, the next order of business will be for you to start figuring out what foods you may want to be putting into your diet. This, of course, is influenced both by your personal desires, as well as the other complexities that may exist with juggling your eating regiment with other household members.

It's important that you document the calorie count for the foods that you choose, which means having accurate food weights, or volumes, and knowing the correct calories for those amounts. Accuracy is very important, as an error here can accidently take you well off course, and this is a major part of your accountability to yourself; the good news is that this all gets fairly easy after you've established a pattern of the foods that you decide to be eating.

There are a few general areas to look at before starting to discuss any specific foods. Most people realize that non-starchy vegetables should be high on your list of foods to eat, because most of those contain fewer calories than meats, starchy foods (including starchy vegetables), and sweets. The most common starchy vegetables we encounter seem to be potatoes, corn and some types of squash. Non-starchy vegetables tend to be things like cauliflower, broccoli, asparagus, cabbage, eggplant, zucchini, lettuce and cucumber. And, then you have your legumes (beans), tomatoes, and others. When you start examining the calories in vegetables, even the starchy vegetables, you realize that intrinsically many don't necessarily contain a huge number of calories, but so often these vegetables are served with butter, cheese sauces and other such things that turn them into high calorie foods. It's okay to eat them that way if they fit into your diet plan, but be sure to honestly account for the extra calories.

Before going further, I want to make clear that I eat meat as a regular part of my diet, and always have. I have great respect for those who are vegetarians and vegans, and I assure you that there are more than an adequate number of weight loss recipes readily available that specifically accommodate those menus. The SparkPeople® website, for example, has a large number of recipes that are specifically oriented to vegetarians, and also ones for vegans. I mention this because the recipe ideas that I offer in the following paragraphs are my own, and many tend to be meat oriented. I want to be very clear that whether a person eats meat, or chooses not to eat meat, is totally irrelevant to the success of this weight loss program.

When it comes to fish, poultry and other meat, clearly fish is the big winner (calorie wise), though some fish like salmon does have a higher fat content, and therefore more calories. If you remove the fat from poultry, which essentially means the skin, and most of the stuff just under the skin, then poultry turns out to be a very good meal choice. Like a lot of Americans I personally enjoy beef and pork (including ham). After doing a fair amount of research I found that as long as you purchase the less fatty cuts of beef, namely those cuts with a minimum amount of marbling fat running through the meat, and then you aggressively trim all of the fat from the meat, it becomes much more diet friendly, at least when eaten in moderate portions.

Many people truly enjoy sweets, including chocolate, pies, cookies and cake. Unless foods like these are sweetened with artificial sweeteners, which is nutritionally unacceptable to many people, the best thing to do with these meal choices, is to limit your consumption to only a bite or two, so that you at least get the taste, but still avoid most of the calories. Your diet survival is not only dependent on your taking in a reduced number of calories, but also on your maintaining your ability to at least have a taste of those things that you truly enjoy. This may sound difficult in the beginning, but I assure you that it's all very easily achievable, especially if you keep your "why" clearly focused in your mind, especially when eating.

As I stated in the beginning, I'm a person who enjoys vegetables. I don't crave sweet foods, and I definitely enjoy the taste of many fatty foods. As I said earlier, I'd choose a hamburger over a piece of pie, every time. I point that out because I won't have too much to say about sweet foods, and when I do eat sweets, I mostly choose artificial sweeteners; my favorite non-calorie sweetener is Stevia, which is natural food extract, but I also sometimes use other artificial sweeteners, too. Some people have some health/nutritional issues with artificial sweeteners, but that's something personal that you'll have to decide for yourself. Natural sweeteners that contain sugar, also all have calories, so if you use them you'll again need to carefully calculate the calories involved. On occasion, I'll also use an Agave sweetener (only because I like it), but the 20 calories a teaspoon, is about equal to any other sugar syrup, so I don't kid myself, I just account for the calories.

Menu Items To Consider

I'll briefly describe a few dishes that I enjoy, but in no way do I intend this to be a cookbook, or anything close to it. In discussing cooking, I'm simply trying to illustrate how with a little effort, enjoyable food with minimal calories, can easily be prepared. In fact, when eaten in moderation, there are a lot of foods that can pretty easily fit within anyone's diet structure.

I love spaghetti type dishes, but I never use premade marinara sauce, as I know that most of those store bought sauces contain added sugar, and more calories than I care to consume. I make my own sauce, and in my case I usually choose to make it a meat sauce, by using very lean ground turkey. This kind of sauce tastes great, and has fewer calories then the premade marinara sauces. Also, I never mix the pasta in with the marinara sauce prior to serving, as I like to be able to keep the pasta serving small, allowing me (calorie wise) to have a full serving of sauce. This same sauce can be used as a base for eggplant parmesan, lasagna, ravioli, chili and even pizza, but keep the pizza crust thin with minimal cheese and toppings. The calories in many of these dishes are almost completely controlled by how much cheese is added and how much pasta you use; so just restrain yourself from putting in too much cheese, and using too much pasta.

Because we just discussed pasta, perhaps we should discuss bread. Garlic bread is a common side dish with pasta, and when we have guests I always serve garlic bread with melted butter, but it is not something I choose to eat myself. For me bread has way too many simple carbohydrate calories, which metabolize just like sugar, so that's a food that I mostly try to skip. Often, I will even order a hamburger at a fast food restaurant, and ask for it with no bun; for me it makes just as nice a meal with lettuce and tomato, than it does the hamburger with bun. I also tend not to use any ketchup or mayonnaise, but will substitute mustard, which is has almost no calories.

I love salads, and I especially like them when they include fresh tomatoes, fresh lettuce and a few shrimp (but that's just my choice). The problem with salads isn't the salad itself; it's the salad dressing that can make it a problem for diet and weight loss. Many salad dressings come in low calorie versions, but be sure to check the actual calories on these low calorie versions, as their idea of low calories usually still seems pretty generous to me. One interesting trick that I learned from someone who belonged to "Weight Watchers®", is to order a salad with the dressing on the side, and then just dip your fork into the dressing before using it to pickup the bite of salad, this way you still get the flavor of the dressing, while consuming less calories. Other salads, like a chef salad, Cobb salad or taco salad, from purely a calorie perspective, are all typically loaded with calories, and you might just as well eat a sensible entrée. If you're eating salads like theses regularly, and doing so to lose weight, it's more than likely that you're just kidding yourself. If you are intent on maintaining an effective weight loss program, be sure that you honestly track your calories.

There are a number of dishes that I like to make that use either lean beef, lean pork, turkey or chicken. Roasting meats are my preference, over frying, as it's a more calorie friendly way to cook. I often place some vegetables around the roasting meat, add a can of broth, and then use the broth/meat drippings as a nice topping for the vegetables, in place of using butter or another kind of sauce.

When it comes to burgers, I almost always use lean ground turkey, or sometimes ground chicken. I almost never use ground beef when cooking at home as it tends to have more calories, and I like the turkey just as well. The turkey, in my opinion, does not barbeque as well as ground beef, so on those occasions I do use lean ground beef. I'm also very careful to watch the ketchup, mayonnaise and especially the barbeque sauce, as they are all loaded with a lot of calories. Pickles, onions and mustard, however, are great with burgers as they have few, if any, calories.

Coleslaw is another popular side dish with burgers, but it has a calorie heavy mayonnaise base, and store bought coleslaw (also used in most restaurants) almost always has sugar added, so it's pretty heavy in calories. If you like coleslaw, and want to watch your calories, it's best to make it yourself.

One of my favorite lunch meals is soup, and if you are someone when enjoys eating soup, you'll find that soup can be a very weight-loss friendly meal. I personally enjoy many of the "Light" soups that are on the market, a 16 ounce bowl has as few as 140 calories, and it makes a nice lunch all by itself. Soups for main meal are a great way to make use of leftovers, too.

Fish is a very calorie friendly food, and there are two fish dishes that I always think of as a soup, but are more technically a stew. The first is Cioppino, which is a wonderful low calorie fish stew that originated in San Francisco, and is considered an Italian-American dish. Bouillabaisse is somewhat similar to Cioppino, and is a traditional French fish stew that originated in the port city of Marseille. Both dishes are delicious, and delicacies often found at many fine dining restaurants. But, don't let that deter you, the Internet has lots of good recipes for both of these great dishes, they can be easily modified to suit your taste, and they aren't that hard to prepare at home.

Mexican food is another very popular kind of food. Mexican food is typically loaded with cheese, flour tortillas (often deep-fried), rice and refried beans. Taco salads, nachos with cheese, and most burritos are very hard to justify from a calorie perspective. Even the simple taco usually contains many more calories than you might suspect. Personally, I love to have a plate of cheese-covered nachos as a treat, but I rarely have it because I find that for me, Mexican food pretty much stays off-limits.

I think it's pretty easy to see that there are some pretty standard "culprits" in the American diet. Foods like anything deep-fried, fatty meats (such as bacon, pork, beefsteak), fatty foods like cheese, butter and peanut butter, whole milk, sugary foods (jellies, syrups, candies and many breakfast cereals), breads, pasta, starch vegetables and more, all are foods that tend to be major calorie "culprits". Of course, it's unrealistic to think that you can, or should, totally avoid these foods; the real challenge is in understanding, and honestly tracking, the amount of these food calories you consume each day. Your personal weight loss program relies on your knowledge of food calories, your willingness to consume them in a sensible fashion, and upon your honest accountability to yourself.

As if the food hurdles outlined above aren't enough, there are also some food condiments, which are not very calorie friendly. Condiments such as mayonnaise, ketchup, barbecue sauce, gravies, other flour-based sauces, butter and cream based sauces, cheese sauces and more, should all be either avoided, or used only in extremely limited amounts. In many respects these kinds of sauces almost become our biggest hazard, in that they can so easily be eaten with otherwise low-calorie foods, and completely blow the dish out of the water with their additional calories.

Obviously we haven't covered every kind of food. The Chinese, Japanese and other oriental dishes can all be wonderful calorie wise, or terrible. All of these have become Americanized with large qualities of deep fat frying, rich calorie laden sauces and so on. If you cook your own, you'll more than likely be much better off. We skipped cereals, deserts and rice dishes too, all of which can be reasonably problematical calorie wise. Another food is eggs, which although the yolk has fat calories, one large egg is only about 59 calories. If you cook them in grease, or put cheese on them like an omelet, you add a lot more calories. Hard-boiled eggs, and poached eggs, are much easier to fit into a calorie conscience diet. Fortunately, it's possible to learn the calories for pretty much everything today, so that's what you're going to have to do for your own favorite dishes.

Getting The Most From What You Eat

Hopefully, I've painted a clear picture that shows you that your weight loss plan is totally up to you including what you eat, how much you eat and when you eat. More important is your accountability to yourself, as you're the "food police" and must enforce your own program. It also requires that you put some serious effort into learning more about the caloric, and nutritional, value of the foods that you decide to eat, because it all boils down to some pretty simple arithmetic. You only have a certain number of calories that you've designated for your daily calorie target, so each time during the day that you choose to eat a calorie laden food you simply must subtract those calories from your daily total, and when you do that, it becomes completely clear where your weight loss program stands at any given time. Pretty much everything in life that's worthwhile, requires effort and dedication, and the success of your weight loss program is no different. With that said, there is some good news, and that is that there're a lot of things that you can eat that taste good, and can easily be included in virtually any diet. So, let's take a look at some of those things that very well might brighten your weight loss day.

Let's talk about some of your weight loss "friends", and we can start with water. Most dietary experts will tell you that drinking eight, 8oz cups of water every day is important for your health, and I'm sure that's true. But, I find one of the nice things about water is that is an excellent solution should your stomach start growling between meals. The digestive process in your stomach, and its acids, more often than not cause those pangs of hunger. They've built up because of past snacking habits, but simply drinking a glass of water will very often make those hunger pangs disappear, and in the process you will have consumed zero calories.

Fruits do contain sugar, but those calories are mostly in limited quantities, making them dieter's good friend, especially for those who enjoy sweets. In fact, if you shop in health food stores, you can usually find fruit jellies that are only sweetened with the sugar from the natural fruit (no sugar added), and used sparingly these makes a really nice treat. There are also a lot of other similar options, so check out your local stores.

There is no doubt that salt and fat laden chips are not at all weight-loss friendly. Pretty much everyone knows that fresh carrots, celery and cucumbers make nice healthy snacks, but on the other hand they are not necessarily popular with a lot of people. And, in that this customized weight loss program is designed specifically for you it's important that it contain foods that you enjoy. One idea I like, which is a bit of a compromise, is to buy the cooked corn tortillas (or better yet bake them yourself), and break them into small chips to snack on. They do have calories, but usually fewer than potato chips, nachos and others, and because the packaging will make it easy to tell how many calories there are in each tortilla, it's pretty easy to control how much you consume. I also like some thin bread sticks that are available locally, 1 stick that's about 10" long and ¼ " around is only 11 calories. Eaten in small bites, it's a nice "crunchy" snack. Learn to be creative in finding lower calorie substitute foods that you still find enjoyable, it will be a major key to building and sustaining your long-term weight loss program.

Another trick that I learned a while back is to substitute mashed cauliflower for mashed potatoes. Now, I'm personally not too much of a cauliflower lover, but I couldn't resist going ahead and trying this dish. Actually, it worked out quite well, and if you cook the cauliflower until it gets mushy, it can easily be mashed, and when seasoned with salt and pepper to your taste, it's surprisingly good. In that I use a zero calorie "I can't believe it's not butter spray®" as a substitute for butter, the dish becomes very calorie friendly. The reason I haven't made this dish more often, is because mashed potatoes are typically not part of our normal diet, but if you like to regularly enjoy mashed potatoes, you may want to try this option, but of course, if you add in gravy, or butter, you also start adding a lot of calories.

I realize that not everybody likes seafood, which to me is a shame because I love it, and it's one of those foods that is both healthy, and typically contains very few calories. There's a lot of seafood that can be baked, broiled, boiled or otherwise cooked in a calorie free method. All of these taste delicious when seasoned only with some nice spices, and perhaps a little lemon juice. Of course, there are a lot of seafood lovers that like to have seafood covered in butter, battered and deep-fried, or with some other sauce, all of which takes away the benefit of the low-calorie seafood. If you have no personal nutritional issue with using the zero calorie "I can't believe it's not butter spray®", the issue of butter flavor is easily solved.

Food Shopping

The last thing that I want to touch on in the section, is food shopping. Once you've done your calorie/nutrition research, and have made your choices as to which foods are going to work best for you, it's time to go shopping. But before you do that there's one more thing that I will again recommend that you do, and that's is to clean out the entire old calorie laden foods from your cupboards, and refrigerator. If you have a friend, family or a neighbor who would enjoy having the food then that's great, otherwise put it out into the garbage. It is simply too great of a temptation to have those kinds of foods easily available, unless it's absolutely essential because of other family members in the household. And, in that case it's best to try to keep those foods separated in a fashion that makes them not easily accessible. Experience has taught me, and probably you too, that one of the hardest parts of any weight loss program is getting it successfully started, and eliminating your temptations is a big positive step in that direction.

The first thing that you're going to want to do is to create a shopping list, as it will help you stay accountable for just buying those foods that you've already decided are acceptable. Supermarkets were among the very first retailers to learn the benefits of marketing impulse foods to shoppers, and they have learned to do it very effectively. Impulse foods are typically displayed at the ends of the food aisles, as well as near the checkout, and they're almost never the healthy foods that you should be buying. You'll also find that the more popular unhealthy foods are the ones typically displayed at eye level, so you'll want to be sure to look both up and down along the shelves, to discover some of the less popular, but healthy food options. For this reason I strongly encourage you to take the time to make a comprehensive shopping list of the foods that you have decided will work for your weight loss program, and simply buy nothing else while at the market.

Whenever possible I like to do a lot of my shopping at health food stores, as they often carry some of the specialty foods that are either low calorie, or even no calorie foods. But make no mistake just because a food is in a health food store does not mean that it's either healthy, or qualifies to be on your food list. There are some phrases that food retailers love to use, like low-fat, fat-free, natural, organic, low calorie, no sugar added, and sugar-free. Not one of these phrases will ensure that any given food will qualify (calorie wise) for your weight loss program. I cannot overstate the importance of doing your research, and in carefully reading the label on all foods before you purchase them. If you wait until you get home to read the label, there's a great likelihood that you will eat the food because you just purchased it, even if it does not meet your criteria. So again, I advise you to take your time, and read every label while you're in the store, before you purchase the food item.

The best time to go shopping is after you've had a meal, shopping while hungry is a very risky thing to do. It's amazing how much better some foods sound to you when you're hungry. When you go food shopping on an empty stomach, you run a serious risk of buying things that you really shouldn't be eating, so it's best to do your food shopping on a full stomach!

Lastly, the supermarket is also an excellent place to do new food research. In the frozen food department in particular, if you'll read the labels carefully you'll find numerous foods that have been prepared to the standards of "Weight Watchers®", and other similar organizations. Although these prepared foods may not be as nutritional, and may not work well for your current menu, they can be really nice to keep in the freezer for an emergency meal, so that you don't get carelessly trapped into eating something with too many calories. You will also find that there are some lower calorie ice creams, or other frozen snacks, that can be attractive calorie wise, and that may make a nice special treat. However, it isn't particularly wise to keep that type of snack readily available in your freezer, especially if you're an individual who is particularly attracted to sweets, as you may be too easily tempted to eat more than you should. Always remember that this weight loss program is for you, and by you, so the choices always remain up to you, just as the results will remain your responsibility, too.

After You Arrive At Your Weight Loss Goal

This book is primarily about weight loss, and how to create your own personal path for successful weight loss. Needless the say, there will come a time when you no longer want to lose more weight. And, as you start approaching your target weight, my recommendation is that you slowly start giving serious thought to what your long-term maintenance diet, and exercise program, is going to look like. Because you built your weight loss program around the foods that you like to eat, and the way that you like to eat, you shouldn't have a tremendous amount of adjustment as you slow to a level weight.

When you fly in an airplane, you're aware that before the plane arrives at the airport, it starts to slow down to speed where it can be easily landed on the ground, and comfortably brought to a safe stop. Think of your diet in the same way, and as you start approaching your target weight begin to make small adjustments in your program. The very final stages of your weight loss program should be one where the rate of weight-loss begins to diminish, and finally your weight is comfortably stabilized at the target that you've chosen.

Because it's your desire to have a long-term weight stabilization program, it's very important that you carefully make your "landing" at a safe and comfortable speed. It's important to recognize that if you've had an ongoing weight issue in your life, then you need to accept the fact that you're going to have to have a life long weight maintenance program, It's really no different than a diabetic who must maintain a life long insulin management plan. If you think that's not the case, then you're doomed to the yo-yo club.

Section VIII
Identify Your Support Group

It's not going to come as a surprise to you that your weight loss success is going to have its challenges. You're decision to head down this path to weight loss success, was an important personal decision. It was a decision you had to make on your own because of all the extremely personal aspects to it, especially the identification of your personal reason "why" you're on this path. You're the only person that sits in judgment of your diet and exercise plan, and the resulting changes in your life. With that said, we are all different, and for many people there may be times when you'll want, and need, the support of others. So, if you feel that you're such a person, then you may wish to take some time to look around in order to find someone with whom you'll feel comfortable sharing your weight loss decision, as later you may wish to ask for their support.

It's important that you identify people that will absolutely be positive, and be unconditionally supportive; they could be your family, your friends and even a coworker. Should you decide to look to others for support, the number of people you choose isn't what's important, though I personally feel the fewer the better, the thing that's really important to you is that you find people who you can absolutely trust, and who you know will be supportive, and encouraging, of your efforts. Even if you only have one person with whom you have this kind of supporting relationship, that's fine as this is all about the quality of support you have, not the quantity. I can say that personally, my only outside support comes from my wife, and that works just fine for me.

There is also other support available too, groups like "Weight Watchers®", neighborhood or community weight loss groups and of course there are numerous Internet based groups available. You may not find some of these groups right away, you may join some and later dropout, and then join others. What matters the most is that if you want support, that you have at least someone you feel comfortable going to, and who will never sit in judgment of your plan, or your progress.

Lastly, the most important person to fully support your weight loss program is you! You need to become your own best friend, and always feel proud of what you doing. Engage yourself, fully and productively, in your weight loss plan, and allow others to see that you have tremendous respect for yourself, and for the weight loss decision that you've made. When others observe your positive demeanor, and your consistent self-confidence, they too will become enthusiastic about what you're are doing, and that will in turn make you even more enthusiastic. Enthusiasm begets enthusiasm.

Section IX
Conclusion

The most important thing that my book can do is to convince you to fully, completely, and specifically identify the true reasons "why" you want to achieve long-term weight loss. *Having your "why" indelibly in your mind all of the time is critically important to your success; in fact this is the biggest single secret for the achievement of your weight loss victory.* If you choose to only search on the surface for your "why", you'll achieve less than what you desire. Although finding your deep-seated "why" is the single most important action that you can take in your weight loss endeavor, there's one more thing that can multiply its effectiveness.

At one time or another, you've probably touched a hot stove, or some other very hot surface, and burned yourself; I think we've all done that. Hopefully when that happened you weren't seriously injured, but just received a painful message that you should be very careful about touching hot surfaces in the future. And, I'll bet that throughout your life, you've always carried that message with you, don't touch the hot stove, yet that still didn't keep you from being around the stove, it just reminds you that you should be careful when you're around it. Think about food as if it were a hot stove, and your weight loss "why" as carrying the message for you to be careful when you're around food. At the point where you are able to always connect your "why" with food, whenever and wherever you're around food, then you'll have your automatic reminder to be cautious about what you eat, and how much you eat. Believe me, your weight loss "why" is your true friend when it comes to your weight, and your "why" will always do it's very best to protect you from the overweight pain that you've endured in the past.

My point is, that to only identify your "why", and then not put it into practical everyday application, is much like having an umbrella, and then not bothering to take it with you in case it rains; it can rain almost anytime, and the umbrella is of no help just sitting in the closet. And, so it is with food, as you can be confronted by food at any time, day or night, and having your weight loss "why" with you is the only way it can protect you. Train yourself to always have your "why" close by in mind, right from the time you get up in the morning until the time you go to bed. Always have it with you whenever you're near food; use affirmations or whatever it takes, but train yourself so that every time you see food, your weight loss "why" will jump out and remind you, to be very careful about what you eat. When you regularly do that, you'll have won your weight loss battle.

You will be amazed how quickly, and easily, everything else will fall into place, when you become completely focused on your deeply rooted true reason "why" you want to lose weight. In fact, I'll go so far as to say, that if you meet with some weight loss setback, or failure, the single reason for this will have been because you had either not clearly discovered your true "why", or that you had not learned to keep it with you for your weight loss protection. Seriously, it's that important! When you make that discovery, and that connection, it will set you free; and then you'll be headed down the exciting road to weight loss success. Suddenly you'll find yourself thinking differently about food, and you'll be focused on your new thin self.

Your personalized weight loss program can be as simple, or as complicated, as you decide to make it. Once you have your key fundamentals in place, and designed in a way that's comfortable for you, you'll suddenly find yourself well on your way. In order to successfully achieve the weight loss that you so desire, you're going to have to put forth a lot of personal effort. The stronger your personal "why", and the closer you keep it to you at all times, the easier the effort will seem; and, the changes that you're making will likely feel as if they're being made without sacrifice on your part. Your ability to maintain enthusiasm, and a positive attitude, along with a consistent willingness to be 100% accountable for your actions, will become your great new best friends. As you achieve your first small successes, they'll create new enthusiasm, make you proud of your accountability, and will build even greater self-esteem.

This program is your own path to weight loss success, and it's a process that will absolutely work, but it's dependent upon your willingness to make a commitment, and to take action on your own behalf. I acknowledge that establishing a deep bond with your "why", and holding total belief in you're your goals, may come slowly; I hope that won't happen, but it could. So no matter what rate of weight loss progress you make, always keep your "why" and your goals with you, as their power will never disappear. No matter how big of a weight loss set back you may encounter, those two best friends will still be there for you.

I know that you can do this, the steps are simple, and the plan allows you to make the choices necessary to customize this plan, and to make the plan yours alone. The time period that you decide upon for losing your weight, as well as for achieving your other weight loss goals, is totally up to you, and you alone. For perhaps the first time in your life you will have a weight loss plan that truly belongs to you, one that you completely believe in, and for which you're totally proud. You'll find that the accomplishment of just the first few steps, will propel your positive attitude to new levels, and your weight loss success will suddenly be going full speed ahead; there's no stopping you now!

Congratulations on your new thin, and healthy self, you deserve all of the recognition and rewards that will flow your way! Please stay in touch (see Appendix below); I'd love to hear about your progress and weight loss victories.

Bon appétit (without the un-needed calories)
"Nothing tastes as good as thin feels"

Section X
Appendix

DISCLAIMER: I'm not a physician, I am not a dietician, I'm not a psychologist, and I'm not an attorney. I, therefore, am not giving any medical, dietary, psychological or legal advice what so ever. What I am, is a person who is simply sharing personal weight loss opinions, and observations. Whenever possible, I tried to simplify things in a fashion that was relevant to this weight loss discussion, so therefore if something was omitted, was less than complete, or was less than accurate, it's because this book simply represents my personal weight loss opinion. Most importantly, if you or those close to you, feel that your personal issues are medically or psychologically of concern, or life threatening in any way, please immediately seek proper professional consultation, and advice, as this book is not intended to provide any such advice.

FREE OFFER! To support your weight loss, I will email you my "Weight Loss Forms". These are simply outlines for various forms that you may wish to use in tracking your own weight loss efforts. These forms will be in a Microsoft Word format, PDF file, or a Microsoft Excel format, so that you can easily customize them to suit your own weight loss program. Please put "Weight Loss Forms" in the subject line.

Contact information
If you wish to contact the author, Lyle Gilbertson, he can be reached by email at: WeightLoss@zobsi.net. All emails will be responded to as quickly as can practically be done.

Websites of Possible Interest
www.SparkPeople.com
www.WeightWatchers.com
www.AllRecipes.com/recipes/healthy-recipes/low-calorie/
www.Food.com/recipes/low-calorie

www.FoodNetwork.com/recipe-collection/low-calorie/index.html
www.MyRecipes.com/low-calorie-recipes/
www.cspinet.org - Center For Science In The Public Interest

Books of Interest
"Start With Why", by Simon Sinek
"Find Your Why and Fly", by John Di Lemme
"Dine Out and Lose Weight", by Michael Montignac
"Eat Yourself Slim", by Michael Montignac
"Sensational Stevia Deserts", by Lisa Jobs
"French Women Don't Get Fat", by Mireille Guiliano